Medical Massage Care's

FSMTB Massage & Bodywork Licensing Examination MBLEx Study Guide

2010 Edition

Philip Martin McCaulay

Medical Massage Care Authority, LLC

Table of Contents

Preface

Medical Massage Care's <u>FSMTB Massage & Bodywork Licensing Examination MBLEx Study Guide 2010 Edition</u> will help massage therapy students pass the Massage & Bodywork Licensing Examination (MBLEx) administered by the Federation of State Massage Therapy Boards (FSMTB). The amount of material in this study guide has approximately the same percentage weights as the content of the FSMTB MBLEx exam: 14 percent on Anatomy & Physiology; 11 percent on Kinesiology; 13 percent on Pathology, Contraindications, Areas of Caution, and Special Populations; 17 percent on Benefits and Physiological Effects of Techniques that Manipulate Soft Tissue; 17 percent on Client Assessment, Reassessment & Treatment Planning; 5 percent on Overview of Massage & Bodywork History / Culture / Modalities; 13 percent on Ethics, Boundaries, Laws, and Regulations; and 10 percent on Guidelines for Professional Practice.

I. Anatomy & Physiology

A. System Structure

Circulation System Structure

Cardiovascular system contents:
- Heart
- Arteries
- Veins
- Capillaries

Pulmonary veins - receives oxygenated blood from the lungs
Left atrium - receives oxygenated blood from the pulmonary veins
Left ventricle - receives oxygenated blood from the left atrium
Aorta - receives oxygenated blood from the left ventricle
Right atrium - receives deoxygenated blood from the body
Right ventricle - receives deoxygenated blood from the right atrium
Pulmonary arteries - receive deoxygenated blood from the right ventricle

Digestive System Structure

Digestive system components:
- Mouth
- Tongue
- Teeth
- Salivary glands
- Esophagus
- Stomach
- Small and large intestines
- Liver
- Gallbladder
- Pancreas

Parts of the small intestine, in order starting with the part leading off from the stomach:
1. Duodenum
2. Jejunum
3. Ileum

Order of the colons in which food passes through the large intestine:
1. Ascending
2. Transverse
3. Descending
4. Sigmoid

Endocrine System Structure

Includes glands such as the hypothalamus, hypophysis, thyroid, thymus, parathyroid, pineal, adrenal, pancreas and gonads

Order of major endocrine glands, starting with most superior / cranial:
1. Pineal
2. Pituitary
3. Thyroid
4. Thymus
5. Pancreas

Pituitary gland – the size of a grape

Integumentary System Structure

Integumentary system - includes sebaceous glands, sweat glands, breasts, the skin, hair, and nails

Serous membranes:
- Pleura - covering the lungs
- Pericardium - covering the heart
- Peritoneum - covering the abdominal organs

Classification of epithelia:
- Stratified - many layers
- Cuboidal - found where absorption or secretion takes place

Glands:
- Ceruminous glands - general term for sweat glands
- Eccrine glands – most common sweat glands
- Sebaceous glands - glands along the shaft of the hair
- Apocrine glands - large glands in the axillary region

The order of the layers of skin from most superficial to most deep:
1. Epidermis
2. Dermis
3. Subcutaneous

Superficial fascia - immediately deep to the skin and covers the entire body
Deep fascia - surrounds muscle bellies

Lymphatic System Structure

Lymphatic system components:
- Lymph vessels
- Lymph nodes
- Lymphoid organs
- Lymphoid tissue
- The spleen
- Tonsils
- Thymus gland
- Bone marrow

Order of major lymph nodes, starting with most superior / cranial:
1. Parotid
2. Thymus
3. Spleen
4. Cisterna chili
5. Iliac
6. Inguinal

Spleen:
- Largest lymphoid organ
- Role in regard to red blood cells

Muscular System Structure

Tendon – the part of a muscle that attaches to bone
Belly - the fleshy part in the middle of the muscle
Contractility - the action of a muscle to shorten and thicken
Origin – usually the proximal attachment of a muscle
Insertion – usually the distal attachment of a muscle

Types of Muscle Tissue:
- Skeletal
- Cardiac
- Smooth - bladder

The muscle tendons that pass by the medial malleolus, in order starting with the most anterior, are tibialis posterior, flexor digitorum, and flexor hallucis.

The gastrocnemius muscle crosses two joints.

Tendons:
- Connect muscle to bone
- Parallel collagen fibers
- Can be taut or slack
- Primarily dense fibrous tissue

Aponeurosis - a broad flat tendon that attaches muscle to bone

Retinaculum - a transverse thickening of connective tissue that straps tendons down

Nervous System Structure

Nervous system parts:
- The brain
- Spinal cord
- Special sense organs

Order of major structures of the central nervous system, starting with most superior / cranial:
1. Cerebrum
2. Cerebellum
3. Medulla
4. Spinal cord

Order of major structures of the brain stem, starting with most superior / cranial:
1. Diencephalons
2. Midbrain
3. Pons
4. Medulla oblongata

Dermatomes:
- Zebra striped pattern
- Sensory segment of the skin supplied by a specific spinal nerve root
- C2 is the posterior part of the skull cap, the most superior
- L5 is the most inferior, at the toes

Reproduction System Structure

Female reproductive system components:
- Ovaries
- Uterine tubes
- Uterus
- Vagina
- Mammary glands

Male reproductive system components:
- Testes
- Penis
- Prostate gland
- Seminal vesicles
- Spermatic ducts

Respiratory System Structure

Respiratory system parts:
- Nasal cavity
- Larynx
- Trachea
- Bronchi
- Lungs
- Diaphragm
- Pharynx

Order of parts of the respiratory system, starting with the upper respiratory tract:
1. Pharynx
2. Larynx
3. Trachea
4. Bronchi

Skeletal System Structure

Axial skeleton - skull, vertebrae, ribs, sternum, and hyoid bone
Appendicular skeleton - shoulder and pelvic girdle, lower and upper limbs

Musculoskeletal system - bones, ligaments, tendons, and joints

Patella – kneecap
Clavicle – collar bone
Femur – thigh bone

Bone Structure:
- Compact bone - little space between tissues
- Irregular bone - larger spaces between cells, producing lighter bones

Endoskeleton - an inside bone support structure

Periosteum - irregular small bony plates found at the end of long bones and in the center of other bones, a connective tissue structure covering bones providing for nutrition, growth, and attachments

Piezoelectric - the quality in which bones deform slightly and vibrate when current passes through them

Endosteum - thin membrane of connective tissue lining marrow cavity of a bone containing cells for growth and repair

Classification of Bones:
- Long bones - the larger bones with a shaft and medullary cavity such as the arm bones
- Flat bones - bones such as the ribs that are less round
- Short bones - the small bones found in the hands and feet
- Irregular bones - complex shaped bones such as the vertebrae
- Sutural bones - the bones found in the skull
- Sesamoid - the round bones embedded in joints and tendons such as the patella

Cranial sutures:
- Squamous suture - the articulation of the parietal and temporal bones
- Sagittal suture - the articulation of two parietal bones
- Coronal suture -the articulation of the frontal and parietal bones
- Lambdoidal suture - the articulation of the occipital and parietal bones

Tarsals - Cuboid, Cuneiforms, Navicular

Carpals - Lunate, Pisiform, Hamate

The foot has 14 phalanges.
The hand has 14 phalanges, 5 metacarpals, and 8 carpals.

Medial longitudinal arch - calcaneus to first metatarsal
Latitudinal arch - first metatarsal to fifth metatarsal

Sinus - an air cavity within a bone
Foramen - an opening in a bone through which nerves pass
Meatus - a tunnel or canal within a bone
The zygomatic bone is the cheek bone.

Ligaments:
- Connect two bones
- Uneven collagen fibers that will remain taut
- Primarily dense fibrous tissue

Deltoid ligament:
- Protects against medial stress to the talocrural joint
- Near the medial malleolus, talus, and navicular

Bursa - a small fluid-filled sac that reduces friction between two structures

Special Senses Structure

Eyes - sight
Ears - hearing
Nose - smell
Mouth - taste
Skin - touch

Urinary System Structure

Order of parts of the urinary system, starting with the part connected to the renal artery and vein:
1. Kidney
2. Ureter
3. Bladder
4. Urethra

Renal calculi - crystallized mineral chunks that develop in the urinary tract

B. System Function

Circulatory System Function

Circulatory system function:
- Helps maintain the body temperature
- Circulation

Systemic circulation - blood unloads oxygen and picks up carbon dioxide
Pulmonary circulation - blood unloads carbon dioxide and picks up
oxygen
Left side of the heart - pumps oxygenated blood to all tissues except the
lungs
Right side of the heart - pumps deoxygenated blood to the lungs

Blood types:
- O negative – universal donor blood type
- AB positive - universal recipient blood type

Digestive System Function

Gastrointestinal system function:
- Gateway for nutrients
- Uses the teeth to break food down into small particles

Gastrin - a hormone secreted by the pyloric area of the stomach and
duodenum

For a client with chronic constipation, stimulate peristaltic contraction
of the large intestine.

Endocrine System Function

Endocrine System Function:
- Secretion of chemicals
- Alters the activity of muscle and alters the activity of the immune
system
- Controls growth
- Produces hormones
- Initiates gradual changes in the body that last a long time
- Helps with the regulation of body fluids, metabolism, energy
production, and the reproductive system

Anterior pituitary gland - secretes human growth hormones

Neuroendocrine interaction - a chemical reaction involving
neurotransmitters and hormones

Integumentary System Function

Skin – the first line of defense for the body

Protection is a function of the epithelia.

Membrane - flat sheet of pliable tissue that covers or lines a part of the body

Epithelial membranes – mucous, serous, cutaneous

Mucous membranes line a body cavity that opens directly to the exterior.

Mucous membranes line the digestive, respiratory, and reproductive tracts.

Serous membranes line a body cavity that does not open directly to the exterior.

Synovial membranes line joints and contain connective tissue but no epithelium.

The skin is a cutaneous membrane.

Lymphatic System Function

Lymphatic system function:
- Defense against infection
- Returns excess fluid
- Produces cells for defense
- Closely associated with the immune system

Muscles move lymph.
Fluid flowing into lymph capillaries is derived from blood plasma.

Immunity:
- Passive immunity - can result from antibodies transferred from the mother to the fetus
- Acquired immunity - not present at birth
- Innate immunity -genetically determined
- Active immunity - produced when an individual is exposed to a foreign organism

Muscular System Function

Muscular system function:
- Skeletal movement
- Moves blood
- Generates heat

Skeletal Muscle:
- Attached to bones by tendons
- Cylindrical muscle fibers
- Striations
- Motor neurons

Cardiac Muscle:
- The heart
- Branched muscle fibers
- Striations
- Intercalated disks
- Autonomic nerves

Smooth Muscle:
- The bladder
- Fusiform muscle fibers
- Autonomic nerves

Muscle Fibers:
- Fast twitch - pale, large in diameter, with few capillaries
- Slow twitch - red, small in diameter, with abundant capillaries

Nervous System Function

Nervous System Function:
- Intelligence
- Memory
- Emotion

Effector organ - carries out the response in the reflex arc

Afferent neuron - receives the signal from the receptor organ in the reflex arc

The pleasure center in the hypothalamus releases feel-good neurotransmitters.

Behaviors such as substance abuse, gambling, eating, and thrill seeking are potentially addictive.

Massage can replace potentially addictive behaviors such as substance abuse and gambling.

Myelin - an electrical insulator in the neuroglia

Peripheral Nervous System – Somatic and Autonomic

Autonomic - controls smooth and cardiac muscle
Somatic - controls skeletal muscle contractions

Autonomic nervous system - sympathetic and parasympathetic

Sympathetic Nervous System:
- Fight or flight
- Function of the autonomic nervous system under sympathetic control:
- Constricted blood vessels
- Increased heartbeat
- Decreased secretion of digestive juices
- Sweating

Parasympathetic Nervous System:
- Rest and digest
- Functions of the autonomic nervous system under parasympathetic control:
- Slow heartbeat
- Increased peristalsis
- Increased secretion of digestive juices
- Breathing more slowly

Reproduction System Function

Reproduction system function:
- Reproduction
- Controls sex hormones
- Controls testosterone secretion

The ovum lives for about 72 hours and the sperm live for about 48 hours. The fertile period is about 120 hours.

Respiratory System Function

Respiratory system function:
- Provides oxygen and removes carbon dioxide
- Initiates gas exchange
- Helps with sense of smell

The structure of a part is related to its function:
Thin air sacs in the lung move oxygen rapidly.

The sternocleidomastoid muscle is considered an accessory muscle of
respiration rather than a primary muscle of respiration.

Skeletal System Function

Skeletal system function:
- Supporting framework that protects organs
- Reservoir for minerals
- Where blood cells are manufactured

Origin - the stationary bone
Insertion - the more moveable bone

The structure of a part is related to its function:
- The bones of the skull protect the brain
- The bones of the finger are loose to allow more movement

Shin splints are pain in the tibia bone.

Special Senses Function

Vitamin A - helps the eyes adjust to darkness, prevents night blindness

Lobes of the cerebral cortex:
- Temporal - auditory and olfactory areas
- Occipital - visual reception
- Frontal - speech and thought
- Parietal lobe - touch

Urinary System Function

Urinary system function:
- Regulates blood volume and blood pressure
- Eliminates waste products
- Conserves nutrients

The structure of a part is related to its function:
A thick bladder lining prevents urine from escaping into the pelvic
cavity.

C. Healthcare Related and Medical Terminology

General Knowledge of Body Systems

The order of the levels of organization in the body, from smallest to largest:
1. Chemical level - contains atoms and molecules
2. Cellular level - contains the basic structural and functional units of an organism
3. Tissue level - groups of cells working together to perform a particular function
4. Organ level – two or more types of tissue
5. System level – combination of organs
6. Body or organismal level - the largest level

Chemical level:
- Atom - the smallest unit of matter that participates in chemical reactions
- Element – substance composed of a single type of atom
- Molecules - two or more atoms joined together

Cellular level:
- Interphase – growth, a cell replicating its DNA
- Mitosis - nuclear division that distributes two sets of chromosomes to two separate nuclei
- Meiosis - reproductive cell division in which the number of chromosomes is reduced by half
- Atrophy - a decrease in the size of cells
- Hypertrophy - an increase in the size of cells without cell division

Organelles:
- Organelles - specialized substances within a cell that have characteristic shapes and perform specific functions such as lysosomes, ribosomes, and centrosomes
- Lysosomes -vesicles filled with digestive enzymes that form the Golgi complex
- Ribosomes – most numerous organelles, where amino acids make proteins

Membrane -a thin flexible sheet of tissue
Cytoplasm – material in the cell membrane that surrounds the nucleus and contains organelles
Golgi apparatus or complex - packaging center of the cell

Microvilli – small fingerlike projections that increase the cell surface area

Matrix - the large central fluid-filled cavity of a mitochondrion, enclosed by the inner mitochondrial membrane

Tissue level:
- Four basic types of tissue in the body: Epithelial, connective, muscle, and nervous
- Epithelial tissue - covers body surfaces and forms glands
- Connective tissue - one of the most abundant tissues in the body that binds together other tissues (blood), protects and supports the body and holds organs together
- Muscle tissue - elongated cells that can use ATP to generate force, generates the physical force necessary for movement
- Nervous tissue - detects changes in condition and responds by generating action potentials

Connective tissue:
- Connective tissue fibers - Collagen, reticular, and elastic
- Collagen - fibers that are very strong and resist pulling forces but are not stiff
- Reticular - fibers that consist of collagen in fine bundles and provide support in walls of blood vessels
- Elastic - fibers that are smaller in diameter than collagen and join together to form a network within a tissue

Cells in connective tissue:
- Fibroblasts – repair injured cells
- Macrophages – cells that search for damaged cells and foreign particles
- Mast cells – cells that develop in bone marrow for releasing chemicals
- Adipocytes - fat cells

Cartilage:
- Fibrocartilage - type of cartilage is rigid and made of dense fibrous tissue, such as the cartilage in intervertebral disks
- Hyaline cartilage - type of cartilage is semitransparent, flexible and insensitive, such as the cartilage in the nose

Organ level:
- Different types of tissues joined together
- Heart, liver, lungs

System level - related organs with a common function

Body or organismal level - largest level including all the body systems and parts

Anatomy:
- Anatomy - structures of the body, literally means to cut up and was first studied by dissection
- Surface anatomy - the study of anatomical landmarks through visualization and palpation
- Regional anatomy - the anatomy of specific areas such as the head or chest
- Gross anatomy - the study of structures that can be examined without a microscope
- Systemic anatomy - the study specific body structures such as the nervous or respiratory systems

Physiology - functions of the body, the study of how body parts work
Histology - the microscopic study of tissues

Three fields of physiology:
- Organizational physiology – the study of the body organization
- Pathophysiology – the study of disease
- Systemic physiology – the study of body systems

Catabolism - the process of breaking down substances and releasing energy
Anabolism - the process of building up potential energy
Metabolism - the sum of all physiological and chemical processes in the body including catabolism and anabolism

Passive transport – transportation of substances without energy
Diffusion -the passive movement of ions from an area of higher concentration to an area of lower concentration
Osmosis – diffusion of water
Filtration - the forcing of fluid across a semipermeable membrane
Carrier-mediated transport – proteins bind to substances to carry them
Active transport – movement of substances that requires ATP energy and uses ion pumps
ATP - adenosine triphosphate, a high-energy compound stored in the body or energy currency

Anatomical Position and Terminology

Proximal - closer to the trunk or point of origin	Distal - situated away from the trunk or midline
External - exterior	Internal - within the body
Superficial - on or toward the surface	Deep - inside or away from the surface
Inferior - lower than or below	Superior - higher than or above
Anterior - in front of or toward the front	Posterior - behind or in the back
Plantar - the sole of the foot	Volar - the palm side of the hand
Lateral -on or to the side	
Dorsal - to the back	Ventral - to the front
Medial - relating to the middle	Peripheral - away from the center
Cephalad - toward the head	Caudad - toward the tail or posterior
Valgus deformity - the ends are bent inward, or bent toward the midline: ><, knock-kneed	Varus deformity - the ends are bent outward, or bent toward the wall: <>, bowlegged

The ulna is medial to the radius.
The skin is superficial to the muscles.
The heart is superior to the liver.
The stomach is inferior to the lungs.
The esophagus is posterior to the trachea.
The sternum is anterior to the head.
The lungs are lateral to the heart.
The ribs are deep to the chest and back.
The ribs are superficial to the lungs.
The phalanges are distal to the carpals.
The humerus is proximal to the radius.

Anatomical position - standing erect and facing forward

Zero position - like anatomical position with the hands facing the body and the forearms in between pronation and supination

In anatomical position, the distal ulna is in the medial wrist and the distal radius is in the lateral wrist.

Anatomical Planes

Frontal Plane (Coronal Plane):
- Divides the body into front and back sections or anterior and posterior portions
- Adduction and abduction occur in the frontal plane

Sagittal Plane:
- Divides the body into left and right sections for a lateral view
- Midsagittal or median plane - divides the body into equal left and right sides
- Medial structures are close to the sagittal plane
- Flexion and extension occur in the sagittal plane

Transverse Plane:
- Divides the body into upper and lower portions
- Horizontal plane or cross-sectional plane
- Cranial or caudal structures are farthest away from the transverse plane.
- Rotation occurs in the transverse plane

Oblique plane:
- Passes through the body at an angle
- Between the transverse plane and either the sagittal or frontal plane

The frontal, transverse, and sagittal planes are at right angles to each other.

Order of the body cavities from the most superior to the most inferior:
1. Cranial cavity
2. Vertebral
3. Thoracic
4. Abdominal
5. Pelvic

Body cavities in the dorsal region:
- Cranial
- Vertebral

Body cavities are in the ventral region:
- Thoracic
- Abdominal
- Pelvic

The spinal cord lies in the vertebral cavity.
The abdominal cavity includes psoas major.

Relation of Body Cavities to Diaphragm:
- The cranial and thoracic body cavities are generally more superior to the diaphragm
- The abdominal and pelvic body cavities are generally more inferior to the diaphragm
- The vertebral body cavity is posterior to the diaphragm

Order of the regions of the trunk from the most superior to the most inferior:
1. Cervical - seven vertebrae, neck
2. Thoracic - twelve vertebrae, chest
3. Lumbar – five vertebrae, loin
4. Sacral - five vertebrae fused into one
5. Coccyx – four vertebrae fused into one

Anterior Regions of the Body:
- Frontal – head
- Temporal – temples
- Cervical – neck
- Deltoid – shoulder
- Axillary – armpit
- Brachial – between elbow and shoulder
- Hypochondrium – lateral abdomen
- Umbilical – navel
- Hypogastric – under stomach
- Patellar – knee
- Femoral – thigh
- Inguinal – groin
- Epigastric – abdomen
- Pectoral – chest

Posterior Regions of the Body:
- Occipital – back of head
- Parietal – top of head
- Mastoid – behind ear
- Cervical – neck
- Scapular – shoulder blade
- Lumbar – lower back
- Sacral - below lower back
- Gluteal – buttocks
- Popliteal – back of knee

D. Tissue Injury and Repair

Length of the phase of healing:
1. Bleeding stops and inflammation occurs - 2-3 days to 2-3 weeks
2. Tissue regeneration occurs - 2-3 days to 6 weeks
3. Remodeling of tissue is completed - 6 weeks to 1 year or longer

Fibroblasts – repair injured cells
Macrophages – cells that search for damaged cells and foreign particles
Scar tissue – formation of fibrous connective tissue after wound is healed
Vitamin C - required for tissue repair, essential for blood clotting

E. Concepts of Energetic Anatomy

The Five Elements – Japanese method based on earth, metal, water, wood, and fire
- Metal - lung and large intestine
- Earth - the spleen and the stomach
- Fire - the heart, small intestine, the pericardium and the triple heater
- Water - the kidney and bladder
- Wood - the liver and gallbladder

Chakras (used in Indian and Hindu healing methods):
- Chakras – the seven centers of the Prana
- Laryngeal - located at the front of the throat
- Frontal - located between the eyebrows
- Root - located at the base of the spine
- Coronal - located on the top of the head

Hara – in Chinese and Japanese methods, the belly

Acupuncture, Acupressure and Shiatsu

Meridians:
- Used in energy manipulation techniques acupuncture, acupressure and shiatsu
- Yin meridians – lung, spleen , heart, kidney, pericardium, liver, conception vessel
- Yang meridians – large and small intestine, stomach, bladder, triple heater, gallbladder, governing vessel
- Stomach meridian -begins at the orbital cavity, ends at the second toe, and is associated with food intake
- Spleen meridian - begins at the great toe, ends in the intercostal space, and is associated with digestion
- Liver meridian - begins at the great, ends at the chest, and is associated with the flow of ki (or qi)
- Kidney meridian - begins at the foot, ends at the thorax, and is associated with the impetus to move
- Small intestine meridian - begins at the little finger, ends at the ear, and is associated with assimilation
- Gallbladder meridian - begins at the head, ends at the toe, and is associated with the flow of ki
- Heart meridian - begins at the axilla, ends in the little finger, and is associated with emotions
- Bladder meridian - begins at the head, ends at the little toe, and is associated with purification
- Large intestine meridian - begins at the first finger, ends in the nostril, and is associated with the process of elimination
- Heart constrictor meridian - begins at the thorax, ends at the middle finger, and is associated with circulation
- Chest meridian - begins in the chest, ends in the thumb, and is associated with the intake of ki
- Triple heater meridian - begins at the middle finger, ends at the eyebrow, and is associated with protection

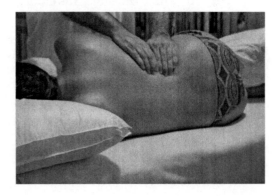

II. Kinesiology

A. Components and Characteristics of Muscles

Phasic muscles:
- Higher percentage of fast-twitch white fibers
- Jump into action quickly and tire quickly
- Usually weaken in response to postural muscle shortening
- Examples – deltoid, biceps brachii

Postural muscles:
- Higher percentage of slow-twitch red fibers
- Relatively slow to respond
- Tend to shorten and increase in tension when under strain
- Examples - erector spinae, soleus

General muscle firing pattern - prime movers, then stabilizers, then synergists
Synergistic dominance - the dysfunction in which muscles compensate for a weak prime mover to produce the movement
Reciprocal inhibition - when a tight muscle decreases nervous stimulation to its antagonist, causing it to reduce activity

Flexors, internal rotators, and adductors are about 25% to 30% stronger than their antagonists.
When a muscle contracts with too much force, it usually overpowers the antagonist group.

B. Concepts of Muscle Contraction

```
Types of Muscle Contractions

Isometric - the length of the muscle does not change, occurs when one
    tries to lift a weight that does not move.
Isotonic - the length of the muscle changes
Eccentric - muscle lengthens
Concentric - muscle shortens
```

Sit-ups, deep knee bends, and squats are eccentric contractions of the biceps femoris.
Eccentric contraction occurs when one lowers a book onto a table.

21

When a jointed area moves into flexion and the joint angle is decreased, the prime mover and synergists concentrically contract.

When a jointed area moves into flexion and the joint angle is decreased, the antagonists eccentrically contract while lengthening.

When a jointed area moves into flexion and the joint angle is decreased, the fixators isometrically contract and stabilize.

Tension can be felt in concentrically short or eccentrically long muscles.

C. Proprioceptors

Proprioceptors:
- Golgi tendon organs
  - Respond to tension and send a signal to the antagonist
  - Protect a muscle from contracting with excess force and speed
  - Send impulses to the central nervous system that lead to muscle relaxation
- Muscle spindles
  - Stretch receptors
  - Respond to sudden and excessive lengthening
- Joint kinesthetic receptors
  - Found in joints
  - Respond to pressure and joint movement

D. Locations, Attachments (Origins, Insertions), Actions and Fiber Directions of Muscles

Rotator cuff muscles – Supraspinatus, Infraspinatus, Teres minor, and Subscapularis

Supraspinatus is on the scapula's anterior surface deep to the upper trapezius.

Infraspinatus is superficial with a medial portion deep to the trapezius and a lateral portion deep to the deltoid.

Teres minor is a small muscle high on the axilla.

Subscapularis is between the subscapular fossa and serratus anterior.

Hip Flexors: Rectus femoris, Gluteus medius, Gluteus minimus, Adductor longus, Adductor brevis, Pectineus, Tensor fascia latae, Psoas major, and Iliacus

The adductors group is medial and the abductors group is lateral.

Hamstrings:
- Biceps femoris, Semitendinosus, Semimembranosus
- The hamstrings group is primarily responsible for flexing the knee

Quadriceps:
- Rectus femoris, Vastus lateralis, Vastus medialis, Vastus intermedius
- The quadriceps group is primarily responsible for extending the knee
- The quadriceps muscles are used when riding a bike

Muscle Attachments

Insertions of Shoulder and Arm Muscles:
- Trapezius - lateral one-third of the clavicle, acromion, and spine of the scapula
- Deltoid - humerus
- Subclavius - clavicle
- Pectoralis minor - scapula
- Pectoralis major - greater tubercle of the humerus
- Subclavius – clavicle
- Latissimus dorsi - lesser tubercle of the humerus
- Serratus anterior - anterior surface of medial border of scapula
- Serratus anterior - anterior surface of medial border of scapula
- Triceps brachii - olecranon process of the ulna

Insertions of Rotator Cuff Muscles:
- Subscapularis - lesser tubercle of the humerus
- Supraspinatus, infraspinatus, and teres minor - greater tubercle of the humerus

Insertions of Forearm and Hand Muscles:
- Biceps brachii -tuberosity of the radius
- Anconeus - ulna
- Pronator teres - radius
- Flexor carpi ulnaris - carpal
- Extensor hallucis longus - phalanx
- Flexor digitorum longus - phalanges

Insertions of Spine and Thorax Muscles:
- Rectus abdominis - cartilage of the fifth, sixth, and seventh ribs and the xiphoid process
- External obliques - the anterior part of the iliac crest, abdominal aponeurosis to linea alba

Insertions of Head, Neck and Face Muscles:
- Sternocleidomastoid - occiput
- Platysma - skin on edge of mandible
- Splenius cervicis - vertebrae
- Oblique capitis inferior - the transverse process of the atlas

Insertions of Pelvis and Thigh Muscles:
- Gluteus medius - greater trochanter
- Gluteus maximus - gluteal tuberosity and IT tract
- Quadratus lumborum - the last rib and the transverse processes of the first through fourth lumbar vertebrae
- Psoas major - lesser trochanter of the femur
- Biceps femoris - head of the fibula
- Piriformis - femur
- Sartorius - the proximal, medial shaft of the tibia at the pes anserinus tendon

Insertions of Leg and Foot Muscles:
- Gracilis - Proximal medial shaft of the tibia at the pes anserinus tendon
- Gastrocnemius - Calcaneus via the calcaneal tendon
- Soleus - Calcaneus
- Tibialis anterior - medial cuneiform and the base of the first metatarsal
- Tibialis posterior - Tarsals and metatarsals

Origins of Shoulder and Arm Muscles:
- Deltoid - Lateral one-third of the clavicle, acromion, and spine of the scapula
- Trapezius - External occipital protuberance, the nuchal line, and C-7 through T-12
- Latissimus dorsi - Vertebrae, the ribs, and iliac crest
- Pectoralis major -clavicle, sternum, and the ribs
- Serratus anterior - the surface of 8 or 9 ribs
- Short head of biceps brachii - Coracoid process

Origins of Rotator Cuff Muscles:
- Supraspinatus, infraspinatus, and teres minor - scapula
- Teres minor - superior half of the lateral border of the scapula

Origins of Forearm and Hand Muscles:
- Flexor carpi radialis - medial epicondyle of the humerus
- Extensor carpi radialis longus - lateral supracondylar ridge of the humerus
- Extensor carpi ulnaris - lateral epicondyle of the humerus

Origins of Pelvis and Thigh Muscles:
- Gluteus medius - external surface of the ilium
- Gluteus maximus - coccyx, sacrum and iliac crest
- Quadratus lumborum - posterior iliac crest
- Psoas major - the bodies and transverse processes of the lumbar vertebrae
- Sartorius - the anterior superior iliac spine (ASIS)

Origins of Leg and Foot Muscles:
- Biceps femoris - the ischial tuberosity and the lateral lip of the linea aspera
- Tibialis anterior - the proximal lateral surface of the tibia

Attachment Sites:
- Nuchal line of the occiput - trapezius and splenius capitis
- Coracoid Process - Pectoralis minor, coracobrachialis, and the biceps
- Medial epicondyle of the humerus - tendons of the wrist and hand flexors
- Greater tubercle of the humerus - supraspinatus, infraspinatus, and teres minor
- Ischial tuberosity - hamstrings, adductor magnus, and the sacrotuberous ligament
- Greater trochanter of femur - gluteus medius, gluteus minimus, and the deep rotator muscles

Locations of Bony Landmarks:
- Medial epicondyle of the humerus - directly medial from olecranon process
- Greater tubercle of the humerus - inferior and lateral to acromion
- Iliac tubercle - posterior to the iliac crest, the boundary of the origins of the tensor fasciae latae and gluteus medius
- Greater trochanter of femur - distal to iliac crest on side of hip
- Tibial tubercle - between the patella and the head of the fibula
- Pes anserinus - medial to the tibial tuberosity
- Tibial tuberosity - distal to the patella on the shaft of the tibia

It is not uncommon for a third peroneal, peroneus tertius, to be present between the patella and the head of the fibula.

Actions of Individual Muscles / Muscle Groups

Actions of Shoulder Muscles:
- Deltoid - abducts, flexes, extends, medially and laterally rotates, and horizontally adducts and abducts the shoulder
- Trapezius - extends, rotates & laterally flexes the head & neck & elevates, depresses, adducts & upwardly rotates the scapula
- Serratus anterior and pectoralis minor - protraction or abduction of the scapula and depression of the scapula
- Trapezius and rhomboids – retraction or adduction of the scapula
- Rhomboid major and minor - adduct, elevate, and downwardly rotate the scapula

Actions of Rotator Cuff Muscles:
- Supraspinatus - abducts the shoulder, can bring the shoulder to 90 degrees
- Subscapularis - medially rotates the shoulder
- Infraspinatus and teres minor (complete synergists) - laterally rotate, adduct, extend, and horizontally abduct the shoulder

Actions of Arm Muscles:
- Triceps brachii - extends the elbow, adducts the shoulder, and extends the shoulder
- Biceps brachii - flexes the elbow, supinates the forearm, and flexes the shoulder
- Brachioradialis - flexes the elbow and assists in pronation and supination of the forearm
- Bicipital aponeurosis - stabilizes the ulna during flexion and supination
- Palmaris longus - flexes elbow
- Abductor pollicis longus – extends and abducts the thumb
- Extensor carpi ulnaris and flexor carpi ulnaris - adduction of the wrist

Actions of Muscles of Head, Neck and Face:
- Sternocleidomastoid - laterally flex and rotate head and neck, flex neck
- Platysma - assist in depression of the mandible

Actions of Muscles of Spine and Thorax:
- Diaphragm - contracts for abdominal inhalation
- External oblique - lateral flexion and flexion of the vertebral column and rotation of vertebral column to the opposite side
- Internal oblique - lateral flexion and flexion of the vertebral column and rotation of vertebral column to the same side
- Internal intercostals - decreases the space of the thoracic cavity
- Semispinalis - extends the vertebral column and head
- Multifidi - rotate the vertebral column

Actions of Muscles of Pelvis and Thigh:
- Biceps femoris - flexes and laterally rotates the knee, extends and laterally rotates the hip, and tilts the pelvis
- Sartorius - flexes, laterally rotates, and abducts the hip; and flexes and medially rotates the knee
- Quadratus lumborum - laterally tilts the pelvis, laterally flexes the vertebral column and extends the vertebral column
- Psoas major - flexes, laterally rotates, and adducts the hip
- Iliopsoas – flexes, laterally rotates, and adducts the hip
- Rectus femoris - flexes the hip and extends the knee
- Gluteus minimus - flexes, extends, medially and laterally rotates, and abducts the hip
- Psoas major - flexes, laterally rotates, and adducts the hip

Actions of Muscles of Leg and Foot:
- Tibialis anterior - inverts the foot and dorsiflexes the ankle
- Tibialis posterior - inverts the foot and plantar flexes the ankle
- Vastus lateralis - extends the knee
- Flexor hallucis longus and abductor hallucis - flex the first toe

The supinator muscle of the right forearm would be used to turn a screwdriver clockwise.

Extension increases the angle between bones.
Flexion decreases the angle between bones.

When the elbow extends, the triceps is the agonist.
When the elbow extends, the biceps is the antagonist.

Radial deviation occurs at the distal radius.
Ulnar deviation occurs at the distal ulna.
Rotation occurs at the radioulnar joint.

A tight and short psoas would decrease the function of gluteus maximus.

Tensor fasciae latae and the adductors would become dominant to compensate for a weak gluteus medius.

If a client complains of difficulty with stair climbing and walking up an incline, the quadriceps femoris is most likely weak.

Muscle Fiber Direction

Triangular	deltoid
Convergent	pectoralis major
Unipennate	extensor digitorum longus
Bipennate	biceps brachii and rectus femoris
Circular	orbicularis oris
Parallel	stylohyoid
Fusiform	digastric
Multi-belly	rectus abdominis

E. Joint Structure and Function

Joint Classification

Synovial - classification of joint has a cavity with fluid

Synovial fluid - thick, lubricating substance secreted by a joint cavity membrane that reduces friction

Synovial joint - freely moving joint allowing movement in one or more planes of action

Joint capsule - connective tissue structure that indirectly connects the bony components of a joint

Types of Synovial Joints

Ball and socket	hip
Saddle	thumb
Pivot	between the axis and atlas
Gliding	between the carpals
Hinge	elbow, knee
Ellipsoidal	wrist

```
┌─────────────────────────────────────────────────────────────┐
│                                                               │
│              Functional Classes of Joints                     │
│                                                               │
│  Diathrosis - freely moveable joint, the joints between the   │
│       tibia and fibula                                        │
│  Amphiarthrosis - slightly moveable joint, the joints         │
│       between the vertebrae                                   │
│  Synarthrosis - immoveable joint, where the bones of skull    │
│       meet                                                    │
│                                                               │
└─────────────────────────────────────────────────────────────┘
```

Synchondrosis - a joint in which a thin layer of hyaline growth cartilage connects two bones such as the first sternocostal joint

Symphysis - a joint with thin layers of hyaline cartilage over bone separated by fibrocartilage such as the two pubic bones

Syndesmosis - a fibrous joint that joins bones with a ligament, cord, or membrane, such as the joint of the tibula and fibula

A suture is a synarthrotic joint in which two bony components are held together by dense fibrous tissue.

Joint Movements:
- Ball and socket joints - allow movement in every plane
- Ellipsoid joints - flexion / extension and abduction / adduction
- Hinge joints -flexion and extension
- Gliding joints - small shifting movements
- Pivot joints – rotation
- Saddle joints – opposition of the thumb and fingers

Flexion and extension - occurs moving forward and backward from the coronal plane in a sagittal direction
Abduction and adduction - occurs moving sideways from the sagittal plane in a coronal direction
Lateral flexion - occurs about a sagittal axis in a coronal direction
Rotation - movement around a longitudinal axis in a transverse plane
Circumduction - only possible with ball-and-socket joints
Gliding - the movement of the scapula an example

Loose-packed position - the unlocked position of a joint
Close-packed position - the locked position of a joint

Joint play - small movements essential for proper joint function

Closed kinematic chains -the positioning in which the movement of one joint moves another joint

Open kinematic chains - the positioning in which a joint is free to move without causing motion at another joint

Arthrokinematics - accessory movements of the articulating surfaces of bones at joint surfaces

Osteokinematics - the movement of bones by action of the muscles

Movement Patterns:
- First class lever:
  - Fulcrum in the middle
  - Lifting the head is an example
- Second class lever:
  - Effort applied at one end and the fulcrum at the other end
  - Like a wheelbarrow
  - Standing on one's toes is an example
- Third class lever:
  - Effort applied at a point between the load and the fulcrum
  - Flexing the arm is an example

F. Range of Motion

Range of motion - the end-to-end distance of a specific joint movement that is structurally possible

Active range of motion - the joint movement that requires the client to use their own energy

Passive range of motion - the joint movement that requires the therapist to move the relaxed client

Anatomic range of motion - the structural limit on the range of motion

Physiologic range of motion - the limit on the range of motion that prevents movement to the point where injury could occur

Pathologic range of motion - the range of motion that could be greater than or less than the normal range of motion

Hypomobility - a joint with a range of motion of less than what it normally would be

Hypermobility - a joint with excessive range of motion, double-jointedness

III. Pathology, Contraindications, Areas of Caution, Special Populations

A. Common Pathologies

Pathology Definitions:
- Pathology - the study of the nature and causes of disease as related to structure and function of the body
- Pathophysiology - the study of functional or physiologic changes in the body that result from various disease processes
- Anatomic pathology - the examination of tissues removed from cadavers or living people for the purpose of studying disease
- Clinical pathology - laboratory medicine

Peritonitis - an inflamed mucous membrane that lines the abdominal cavity

Crohn's disease - a progressive inflammatory condition that may affect any part of the GI tract

Hernia - a hole or rip in the abdominal wall or inguinal ring through which the small intestine may protrude

Emphysema - results in a decreased ability to exhale, with the diaphragm and intercostals not able to work efficiently

Tuberculosis - a highly contagious airborne disease from a bacterial infection that usually begins in the lungs

---

Lateral epicondylitis - tennis elbow, caused by repetitive extension of the wrist or pronation and supination of the forearm

Medial epicondylitis - golfer's or pitcher's elbow, caused by repetitive flexion of the wrist as in throwing

---

Adhesive capsulitis - frozen shoulder

Tendonitis - inflammation of a tendon
Tenosynovitis - inflammation of a tendon sheath

Dislocation - the displacement of bones of a joint

Subluxation - the partial displacement of the bones of a joint, such as the popping sound of the temporomandibular joint

---

Torticollis – tilting of head, caused by spasm in sternocleidomastoid (SCM) muscle

Whiplash – Cervical acceleration-deceleration injury

Lordosis - an overdeveloped lumbar curve
Kyphosis - overdeveloped thoracic curve

Scoliosis - a lateral curvature of the spine
Gibbus - an angular deformity of a collapsed vertebra
List - lateral tilt of the spine

Carpal tunnel syndrome – median nerve of the brachial plexus injured by compression through the carpal tunnel

Injury to ulnar nerve – loss of function of wrist and fingers

Tinnitus – ringing in the ears

Plantar fasciitis – pain and inflammation of the plantar fascia, the area from the calcaneus to the metatarsals on the plantar side of the foot

Jock itch - Tinea cruris, fungal infection on groin area
Athlete's foot – fungus on feet and toes

Sprain – tears to ligaments
Strain – injuries to muscles

Rickets - mainly caused by a Vitamin D deficiency
Scurvy - caused by a Vitamin C deficiency

Osteochondritis dissecans - a form of necrosis in which the cartilage and adjacent bone separate from the bone itself
Osteonecrosis - also known as ischemic necrosis in which the blood supply to a bone is diminished or cut off
Osteogenesis imperfecta - a developmental problem in which the bones are deformed and fragile as a result of demineralization

Legg-Calve'-Perthes disease - degeneration and necrosis at the head of the femur
Scheuermann's disease - caused most commonly by necrosis or inflammation of a bone or disk in the thoracic vertebrae
Spina bifida - a developmental problem in which the vertebral arches do not fuse into the spinous processes

Lou Gehrig's disease - a progressive skin condition that destroys motor neurons in the spinal cord

Arteriosclerosis - arteries become inelastic and brittle

Lupus - a chronic autoimmune disease in which antibodies attack various types of tissue throughout the body

Myositis ossificans - the growth of a calcium deposit in soft tissues, which is always a local contraindication for massage

Ankylosing spondylitis - a rheumatoid inflammatory disorder in which spinal ligaments ossify

Spondylosis - the formation of bony spurs

Spondylitis - the inflammation of more than one vertebra

Spondylolisthesis - the moving forward of one vertebra onto another

Medical Terminology:
- Pathology - the study of disease
- Health - a condition in which all functions are normally active and a state of complete well-being
- Inflammation - characterized by redness, swelling, heat, and pain
- Vasodilatation - the widening of the blood vessels
- Fibrosis - the formation of scar tissue
- Phagocytosis - immune response process to destroy foreign cells
- Hemostasis - the body's automatic response to stop blood loss
- Atrophy - the decreasing size of tissue
- Hypertrophy - the increase in the size of cells without cell division
- Systemic - refers to the body as a whole
- Trauma - a physical injury or wound caused by external force or violence
- Clinical - founded on actual observations and treatment
- Ambulatory - able to walk or not confined to bed
- Anomaly - a deviation from normal

Etiology of Disease:
- Etiology - the study of all factors involved in causing a disease
- Degenerative – a deteriorating disease involving the breakdown of tissues
- Congenital - a disease present at birth
- Idiopathic - a disease with no known cause
- Exacerbation - the increase in the severity of a disease

Signs and Symptoms of Disease:
- Signs of a disease - evidence of a disease as observed by a health professional
- Symptoms of a disease - the described problems of a disease as described by a patient

Modes of Contagious Disease Transmission (e.g., Blood, Saliva):
- Infectious - capable of being transmitted with or without contact
- Opportunistic pathogens - organisms that cause disease only when immunity is low
- Viral - caused by a pathogen that can grow after infecting a host cell
- Fungal - disease caused by molds or yeast
- Bacterial - caused by tiny cells that secrete toxins, eat body cells, or form colonies
- Epidemic - an infectious disease that attacks many people at the same time
- Pandemic – a widespread epidemic
- Breast milk - likely to be a mode of HIV transmission
- Saliva – not likely to be a mode of HIV transmission

Syndrome - a group of signs and symptoms that identify a condition
Prognosis - expected outcome of a disease
Diagnosis - categorization of a disease by a licensed medical professional

Factors that Aggravate or Alleviate Disease (e.g., Biological, Psychological, Environmental)

Biological rhythms:
- Internal periodic timing components of an organism
- Ultradian rhythms - repeat themselves every few hours
- Circadian rhythms - on a 24-hour clock
- Seasonal rhythms - repeat themselves annually

Entrainment - the tendency for oscillating bodies to move in a synchronized, harmonic manner, the coordination or synchronization to a rhythm

Homeostasis - the relative constant state maintained by the physiology of the body maintained by the sympathetic and parasympathetic systems working together
Conservation withdrawal - like hibernation
Toughening/hardening - the reaction to repeated exposure to stimuli that can explain the autonomic reaction to massage

Psychological Healing Process

Therapeutic applications are generally the most acceptable methods to strengthen the healing process.

Pain:
- Pain - an unpleasant subjective sensation
- Chronic pain - an unpleasant feeling that lasts over 6 months
- Somatic pain - a short lived and localized unpleasant feeling
- Visceral pain - an unpleasant sensation from an internal organ
- Referred pain - chest pain from a heart attack is an example
- Phantom pain - pain from an amputated limb
- Acute pain - temporary pain after an operation
- Intractable pain - persistent chronic pain

Principles of Acute versus Chronic Conditions:
- Acute - a disease of short duration, an injury or disease that is a short-term condition that resolves through normal healing processes and care
- Chronic - a disease of long duration, a disease that shows either little change or slow progression

Inflammation or inflammatory response:
- Heat
- Redness
- Swelling
- Pain

A tissue injury could cause inflammation.

Fractures:
- Incomplete fracture - a break that does not go across the entire bone
- Compound or open fracture - a break in the skin and torn soft tissues, where the bone protrudes through skin
- Simple or closed fracture - a break in a bone that does not break the skin or injure soft tissue
- Spiral fracture - a break in which the bone is twisted apart
- Comminuted fracture - more than one fracture line, with several fragments resulting and much soft tissue damage
- Greenstick fracture - an incomplete break in the bone causing it to split, common in children
- Depressed fracture - the bone in skull being driven inward
- Stress fracture - a crack in the bone often caused by repeated mechanical stress and strain
- Impacted fracture - the broken ends of bone being jammed into each other

Five stages of acute fracture healing:
1. Hematoma formation
2. Cellular proliferation
3. Callus formation
4. Ossification
5. Remodeling

Response of the Body to Stress

General adaptation syndrome in response to stress (alarm, resistance, exhaustion):
1. First stage – Alarm, the fight-or-flight response triggered by the sympathetic nervous system
2. Second stage – Resistance, long-term metabolic adjustments occur
3. Third stage – Exhaustion, vital systems collapse

Effects of Physical and Emotional Abuse and Trauma:
- Trauma - the result a violent or disruptive action or a severe emotional shock
- Posttraumatic stress disorder - the re-experiencing of flashback memory
- Detachment - the vague uneasiness when a client does not remember the details of abuse
- State-dependent memory - the manner in which abuse is recalled

Psychological and Emotional States (e.g., Depression, Anxiety, Grief):
- Anxiety - disorder relating to exaggerated irrational fears
  - Anxiety is characterized by rapid shallow breaths that require the use of the accessory muscles of inspiration
- Depression - mood disorder that can result in feelings of hopelessness
- Stress - a stimulus that causes an imbalance

Stress Management and Relaxation Techniques

Stressors - internal perceptions or external stimuli that demand a change in the body
Self-concept - one's opinion of one's self
Denial - a way of coping with stress by ignoring stressors
Emotions - feelings driven by thoughts
Behavior - what we do in response to feelings
Defense measures - the way the body responds to stressors
Posttraumatic stress disorder - the re-experiencing of flashback memory or state-dependent memory
Trauma - what occurs as a result of physical injury by violent or disruptive action

B. Contraindications

Contraindications:
- Thrombophlebitis
- Deep vein thrombosis
- Hematoma
- Acute dermatitis
- Osteomyelitis
- Erysipelas
- Aneurysm
- Lice

Local contraindication:
- Acne
- Bunion
- Cyst
- Open wound
- Warts

Contraindicated in the acute stage:
- Bronchitis
- Herpes zoster
- Gastroenteritis
- Influenza
- Meningitis

Generally indicated for massage:
- Sprains
- Chronic fatigue syndrome
- Bell's palsy
- Joint stiffness
- Irritable bowel syndrome
- Bulimia
- Plantar fasciitis

Leukemia is indicated for massage for people who have survived the condition for five years.
While HIV can be indicated for massage at all stages, it is a systematic contraindication for circulatory massage.

C. Areas of Caution

Nerves:
- Femoral nerve - pierces the psoas major, inguinal triangle
- Greater occipital nerve - pierces the trapezius
- Axillary nerve - teres major, teres minor, long head of the triceps and humerus
- Radial nerve - supinator and lateral head of the triceps, lateral epicondyle of the humerus
- Ulnar nerve – between the medial epicondyle of the humerus and the olecranon process, hand and wrist flexors
- Tibial nerve - popliteal fossa
- Vagus nerve - the heart, lungs, kidneys, and the gastrointestinal tract
- Peroneal nerve - would become entrapped from pressure on the back of the knee
- Sciatic nerve - passes through the hip at the ischial tuberosity and greater trochanter of the femur

> Endangerment site - an area where nerves and blood vessels could be compressed

Endangerment Sites:
- Posterior triangle of the neck – the sides are the SCM, clavicle, and trapezius, includes the subclavian artery and the brachiocephalic artery
- Anterior triangle of the neck – the sides are the SCM, mandible, and trachea, includes the jugular vein and carotid artery
- Sciatic notch - includes a nerve under the piriformis muscle
- Axillary area - the cephalic vein and the nerves of the brachial plexus
- Inguinal triangle - sartorius, adductor longus, the inguinal ligament, and the femoral nerve
- Umbilicus area - includes the aorta
- Twelfth rib, dorsal body - includes the location of the kidney
- Area of the sternal notch and anterior throat - includes the nerves and vessels to the thyroid gland and the vagus nerve
- Popliteal fossa - tibial nerve
- Brachial plexus - C5 to T1, scalenes, clavicle
- Carotid artery - close to the SCM, splenius capitis, trapezius, and scalenes

D. Special Populations

Effects of Life States:
- Adolescence:
  o Homeostasis most optimal
- Senescence:
  o The process of growing old or the period of old age
  o Increased incidence of autoimmune diseases
  o The skin hardens

Atrophy - the wasting effect of advancing age
Stages of lifecycle - the physiological mechanics of aging

Stages / Aspects of Serious / Terminal Illness:
- Malignant neoplasia - Cancer
- Malignant melanoma - an aggressive form of cancer that spreads through the lymph nodes
- Irregular borders - a feature of melanoma but not a mole
- Benign - nonmalignant or not progressive
- Malignant - growing worse
- Metastatic - the spreading or change in location of a disease
- Anaplasia - the reproduction of abnormal cells that fail to mature into specialized cell types
- Hyperplasia - uncontrolled cell division, abnormal tissue growth from uncontrolled cell division
- Neoplasm - a tumor resulting from hyperplasia

Massage is appropriate for terminally ill clients.
When massaging clients with a terminal illness, the goal is to provide comfort.

Sunshine adds to the risk of skin cancer.

Hepatitis B is 100 times more contagious than HIV.
The favorite target of HIV is the T4 cell.

Weight bearing exercise is most beneficial for osteoporosis.
Atrophy is the last stage of osteoarthritis.

A client with hypothyroidism most likely needs a warm room temperature to be comfortable.
A therapist would need to postpone a massage for an athlete if the athlete has heat exhaustion.
Barrier free access is required for physically challenged individuals.
A client with cystitis would require frequent bathroom breaks.

E. Classes of Medications

Topical anesthetics – use of thermal properties to temporarily overwhelm sensors and decrease sensation to an area
Analgesics - non-narcotic pain relievers and narcotics
Antineoplastics - cancer treatment agents
Anti-inflammatory - reduce swelling and pain
Antibiotics - treat a bacterial infection
Antihistamines - allergies
Antidepressants – mood altering, might be used to help someone stop smoking

Prescription Medication

Cardiovascular medications:
- Calcium channel blockers
- Antiarrhythmics
- Diuretics
- Cardiac glycerides
- Anticoagulants
- Antihyperlipidemics
- Antianginals
- Vasodilators
- Antihypertensive agents
- Beta blockers

Respiratory medications:
- Antitussives
- Expectorants
- Decongestants
- Bronchodilators
- Antihistamines

Anti-inflammatory medications:
- NSAIDs
- Adrenocorticosteroids

Gastrointestinal medications:
- Anticholinergics
- Antiulcer medications

Hormones:
- Antidiabetic medications
- Estrogens
- Progesterones
- Androgens
- Steroids
- Thyroid medications

Anti-infectives:
- Antibodies
- Antivirals
- Antifungals
- Anthelmintics
- Scabicide
- Pediculicide

Central nervous system medications:
- Tranquilizers
- Antidepressants
- Amphetamines
- Adrenergic medications
- Antianxiety medications
- Antipsychotics
- Anticonvulsants
- Antiparkinson agents
- Sedatives
- Tranquilizers

Implications for massage for a client taking vasodilators and antianginals - the medication may increase the effect of the massage

Implications for massage for a client taking beta blockers and calcium channel blockers - these drugs may distort the effect of the massage, the client may be susceptible to cold, massage may help with constipation, the blood-pressure lowering effect may result in dizziness, and the medication may result in dizziness after the massage

Implications for massage for a client taking antihypertensives and diuretics - the client may be susceptible to cold, the medication may result in dizziness after the massage, and massage may help with constipation

Implications for massage for a client taking cardiac glycosides - stop the massage if the heart rate slows to below 50 beats per minute

Implications for massage for a client taking anticoagulants - avoid massage methods that can lead to bruising, including compression

Implications for massage for a client taking thyroid medications - changes in stress level may affect the dose

Implications for massage for a client taking anti-inflammatory medications - avoid techniques that could cause inflammation, feedback mechanisms are not accurate, the massage could reduce muscle spasms

Implications for massage for a client taking anticholinergics and narcotics - the relaxation effects of the massage may be altered

Implications for massage for a client taking antiulcer medications - the stress reduction capacity of massage may enhance the effectiveness

Implications for massage for a client taking antidiabetic medications - changes in stress level may impact the dose, the client's physician should monitor the dose, do not provide vigorous massage

Implications for massage for a client taking sex hormones - blood clotting abilities may be changed, the medication may increase fluid retention, and emotional states may fluctuate

Implications for massage for a client taking steroids - changes in stress level may impact the dose, the client's physician should monitor the dose, avoid massage methods that may produce inflammation

Implications for massage for a client taking antihyperlipidemics - occasional muscle and joint pain can occur, the medication may result in dizziness after the massage, and massage may help with constipation

Implications for massage for a client taking anti-infectives - avoid exposing the client to a cold

Implications for massage for a client taking antineoplastics - work under the direct supervision of the client's physician

Implications for massage for a client taking respiratory medications - avoid heat hydrotherapy, the client may be dizzy after the massage, the massage could produce a skin reddening

Implications for massage for a client taking analgesics - watch for bruising, pain perception is inhibited, massage can help with constipation

Implications for massage for a client taking central nervous system medications - massage can increase or decrease the impact of the medication, work with supervision from the physician, massage can help with constipation

Recreational Drugs:
- Recreational drugs impact the hypothalamus by interacting with feel-good neurotransmitters
- Recreational drugs deplete or inhibit the natural production of feel-good transmitters in the hypothalamus
- Depressants such as alcohol block dopamine and norepinephrine

Herbs:
- Peppermint - used for coughs and inflammation of the pharynx
- Ma-huang – ephedra, used for asthma and hay fever
- Lavender - calming scent
- Aloe - used to heal burns
- Eucalyptus - used for coughs

Natural Supplements:
- Saw palmetto - herbal supplement used for urination problems
- Ginkgo - used for memory problems
- Bee pollen - an example of a non-herbal supplement
- Melatonin - a peptide hormone produced by the pineal gland that influence sleep-wake cycles
- Ginseng - used for improving physical stamina
- St. John's Wort - used for mild depression
- Chamomile - used for skin inflammation
- Camphor - used for warts and cold sores
- Brewer's yeast - used for the common cold

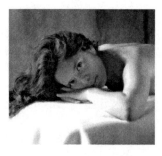

IV. Benefits and Physiological Effects of Techniques that Manipulate Soft Tissue

A. Identification of the Physiological Effects of Soft Tissue Manipulation

Physical effects of massage:
- Increases metabolism
- Hastens healing
- Relaxes and refreshes muscles
- Improves function of lymphatic system
- Helps prevent and relieve muscle cramps and spasms
- Improves circulation of blood and lymph
- Improves delivery of oxygen and nutrients to cells
- Enhances removal of metabolic waste

Effects of Massage on the Muscular System

Petrissage or kneading and compression create a pumping action
Forces venous blood and lymph outward
Brings fresh supply of blood to muscles
Aids in removal of metabolic waste
Helps nourish tissues
Prevents and relieves stiffness and soreness of muscles
Restores muscles fatigued by work or exercised more quickly
Heals injured muscle tissue more quickly
Reduces connective tissue buildup and scarring
Releases fascial restrictions
Reduces thickening of connective tissue (hyperplasia)
Allows more flexibility
Allows easier, pain-free movement
Improved posture
Friction massage reduces adhesions and excessive scarring

Passive joint movement:
- Joints moved with no resistance or assistance from client
- Increases circulation of blood and lymph
- Nourishes the skin
- Relaxes and lengthens muscles, sooths nerves
- Lubricates the joints

43

Active joint movement:
- Muscles resisted or assisted by client
- Beneficial effects similar to exercise

Effects of Massage on the Cardiovascular System

Affects quality and quantity of blood
Dilates blood vessels
Increases red blood cell count
Increases white blood cell count
Increases platelet count
Increases stroke volume
Decreases heart rate and pulse rate
Systolic stroke volume increased
Reduces ischemia
Increases oxygen saturation in blood
Stimulates release of acetylchlorine and histamine for vasodilation

---

Massage movements that affect blood and lymph channels:
- Stroking
  - Light stroking – instantaneous temporary dilation of capillaries
  - Deep stroking – lasting dilation and flushing of massaged area
- Light percussion – causes contraction of blood vessels, which tend to relax as movement continued
- Friction – hastens flow of blood through superficial veins, increases permeability of capillary beds, and increased flow of interstitial fluid
- Petrissage or kneading – stimulates flow of blood through deeper arteries and veins
- Light massage – enhances lymph flow and reduces lymphedema
- Compression – produces a hyperemia or an increase in amount of blood stored in muscle tissue

---

Effects of Massage on the Nervous and Endocrine Systems

Reduces cortisol levels
Increases serotonin and dopamine levels
Increases secretions of endorphins and enkephalins
Reduces pain

Stimulating massage techniques:
- Friction – light rubbing, rolling, and wringing
- Percussion for a short period – light tapping and slapping (prolonged percussion tends to anesthetize the local nerves)
- Vibration – shaking and trembling

Sedative massage techniques:
- Gentle stroking
- Light friction and petrissage (kneading)
- Holding pressure – ischemic compression

Effects of Massage on the Skin

Reduces superficial keloid formation
Stimulates sweat (sudoriferous) and oil (subcutaneous) gland activity
Friction and stroking movements heighten blood circulation
Slight reddening and warming of the skin
Nutrition to the skin is improved

Physiological effects of massage:
- Organic processes of the body
- On cellular, tissue, or organ system levels
- Activation of the parasympathetic nervous system
- The release of endorphins

Categories of physiological effects of massage:
- Reflexive methods – indirect responses to touch
- Mechanical methods – direct physical effects

Mechanical Effects of Massage

The result of the application of physical forces such as bending, compression, stretching, shearing, broadening, and vibration of tissues
Venous return
Lymph flow
Breaking adhesions

Reflexive Effects of Massage

The result of pressure or movement on one part of the body having an effect in another part
Stimulation of the nervous and endocrine systems
Muscle relaxation
Increased mental clarity
Pain reduction
Normalizing system function

Mind-body Effects of Massage

The result of the interplay of body, mind, and emotions in health and disease processes
Anxiety reduction
Relaxation response

Effects of massage that can be processed through the autonomic nervous system (ANS):
- Sympathetic activation and stress
- Mostly reflexive effects
- Parasympathetic patterns and conservation withdrawal
- Entrainment
- Body/mind effect - involves an altered state of consciousness
- Toughening/hardening
- Placebo effect - involves the influence of the treatment itself

Sympathetic stimulation:
- Accelerated heart rate
- Blood diverted to muscles
- Elimination and digestion are inhibited
- Adrenal secretions of epinephrine/adrenaline and norepinephrine increased
- Sweat glands activated
- Body more alert and attentive
- Initially massage alerts sympathetic nervous system
- Pre-event sports massage or 15-minurte chair massage stimulates the body

Parasympathetic stimulation:
- Reduced heart rate
- Increased digestion and elimination
- Increased circulation to internal organs
- Relaxation/restorative response
- Longer relaxing massage

Homeostasis – maintained by the sympathetic and parasympathetic nervous systems working together

Effects of massage that can be processed through the somatic nervous system:
- Reduction of impingement
- Neuromuscular mechanisms
- Hyperstimulation analgesia
- Counterirritation

It usually takes 10 to 15 minutes before massage activates the parasympathetic nervous response.

Inactive muscles benefit greatly from massage because oxygen and nutrients are delivered.

Cortisol is decreased as one of the effects of massage.

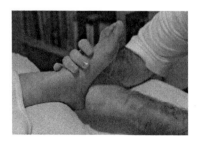

B. Psychological Aspects and Benefits of Touch

Psychological effects of massage:
- Relieves fatigue
- Reduces tension and anxiety
- Calms the nervous system
- Promotes a sense of relaxation and renewed energy
- Rebuilds positive self-image and sense of self-worth
- Reduces aversion to touch for sexual abuse victims
- Reduces depression and anxiety
- Reduces stress
- Promotes relaxation and mental alertness
- Helps client become aware of where there is muscle tension

C. Benefits of Soft Tissue Manipulation for Specific Client Populations

Conditions that can benefit from massage:
- Alzheimer's disease
- Anemia
- Asthma
- Attention deficit hyperactivity disorder
- Autism
- Burn victims
- Cancer (conditionally)
- Cerebral palsy
- Chronic fatigue syndrome
- Constipation
- Diabetes
- Eating disorders
- Fatigue
- Fibromyalgia
- Headaches
- High blood pressure
- Injuries
- Insomnia
- Joint immobility
- Low back pain
- Lung disease
- Lymphedema
- Multiple sclerosis
- Muscle spasms
- Nerve entrapment
- Pain in shoulders, neck, back, and joints
- Poor circulation
- Pregnancy and postpartum
- Premenstrual syndrome
- Psychiatric patients
- Rheumatoid arthritis
- Skin conditions such as mild dryness
- Stress, tension, and anxiety
- Temporomandibular joint dysfunction

Groups that can benefit from massage:
- Individuals with HIV
- Hospitalized and hospice patients
- Infants

Pregnancy massage:
- Use light effleurage and supine or side-lying position
- Beneficial for back strain and strained leg muscles
- Prone position (face down) uncomfortable and dangerous in second and third trimesters
- Avoid massaging abdomen
- Avoid deep tissue massage and percussion
- Toxemia (pre-eclampsia) contraindicated

Massage supports the treatment of addictive behaviors:
- Stimulates the release of feel-good neurotransmitters
- Replaces destructive manner of mood alteration with constructive method
- Stimulates the release of feel-good hormones

Massage for the critically ill:
- Not contraindicated
- Purpose is to provide comfort, pleasure, and relaxation
- Helps control pain
- Improves mobility
- Reduces isolation
- Allows for a more positive outlook
- Touch, slow and gentle stroking, and energy work are most common
- Length of session may be abbreviated
- Techniques that stir up circulation and stir up wastes may not be appropriate

Working with HIV-Infected Individuals:
- HIV is a virus that can destroy the immune system
- An HIV-infected person with a low T-cell count and an opportunistic infection has AIDS
- The HIV virus is found in blood, semen, vaginal fluids and mother's milk
- The HIV virus is rarely found in saliva

Guidelines for Massaging Persons with Cancer:
- Take a complete medical history
- Consult the physician
- Develop a treatment plan
- Use light to moderate pressure and shorter sessions
- Deep massage is contraindicated
- Massage in the area of the tumor or lymph lodes is contraindicated
- Avoid circulatory massage
- Avoid massage in case of fever
- Be aware of surgery concerns
  - Increased chance of blood clots, hemorrhage, and thrombosis
  - Avoid massage on site of incision
  - Massage on lower limbs contraindicated post-surgery
  - Scar massage may be started after 4 to 6 weeks with doctor approval
- Consult physician for clients receiving chemotherapy

D. Soft Tissue Techniques

Effleurage

Swedish massage
Gliding, slow strokes with even pressure
The best transition stroke
Best for applying lubricant
Not the best stroke for ticklish clients
Improves health of ischemic tissues
Good for clients with insomnia
Nerve stroke - a type of superficial effleurage
Knuckling
Deep effleurage - best for local deep massage of soft tissue
Gliding clockwise strokes on the abdomen if a client has chronic constipation
Ethereal body or Aura stroking – long, smooth strokes
Feather stroking – light pressure with long flowing strokes
Beneficial for clients with edema
Reduces high blood pressure
Best stoke for the beginning and end of a massage
Most appropriate stroke for the elderly

Petrissage

Swedish massage
Kneads soft tissue
Kneading – lifts, squeezes and presses tissues
Fulling - spreading the muscle belly outward, away from the midline
Skin rolling
Uses a grasping and lifting action to pull tissue from bone
Uses a rhythm of about one stroke per second
Best stroke for removing waste
Heat is produced when muscles are kneaded
Breaks up adhesions in muscle belly
Variations include one-hand, "C" hand position and "V" hand position

Tapotement

Swedish massage
A fast rhythmic stroke, rapid striking movement
Best stroke for bronchitis and loosening congestion
Tones weak muscles
Cupping
Percussion
Hacking
Slapping
Tapping – appropriate for the face
Beating
Pummeling – using loose fists
Not appropriate for pregnant clients

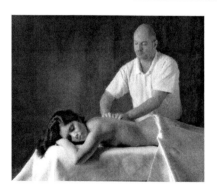

Friction

Swedish massage
Addresses adhesions in tendinous tissue, increases joint flexibility
Gives best information about connective tissue
Superficial friction - a variation of light effleurage
Friction or deep effleurage – best for breaking up areas of hard tissue
    build up or fibrosis
Deep fiber friction - uses localized pressure to break up adhesions
Circular friction – best stroke for the mandibular region
Rolling – for massaging the arms and legs
Wringing – back and forth movement of both hands
Cross fiber friction (transverse friction):
- Reduces scar tissue
- Stretching or pulling
- Effective for reducing adhesions during sports massage
- More effective without oil
- Appropriate for treating tendonitis
- Rehabilitation for athletic injuries

Vibration

Swedish massage
High frequency hand movements
Involves a slight trembling of the hand
Reduces intensity of deep tissue techniques
Trembling, jostling, shaking
Rocking – push and release movement
Rocking the leg would create mobility of hip joint

Compression

Applies pressure to soft tissues to squeeze them together without any slip
Involves temporarily stopping blood flow to an area, then releasing to
    allow greater blood flow
Effective for applying pressure during sports massage
Appropriate for massaging the intercostals

Muscle Energy Techniques:
- Muscle Energy Technique (MET) - another name for proprioceptive neuromuscular facilitation (PNF), including reciprocal inhibition and post isometric relaxation, an assisted stretching technique that increases flexibility
- Reciprocal inhibition (RI) - client contracts the antagonist to the target muscle, reduces muscle cramping
- Direct manipulation (DM) - a PNF technique in which the muscle spindles and Golgi tendon organs are used to relax a hypertonic muscle
- Post-isometric contraction (PIR) - a proprioceptive neuromuscular facilitation (PNF) technique that uses active movement to lengthen the muscle
- Positional release (PR) - a PNF technique involves holding and waiting for the nervous system to trigger relaxation, strain / counterstrain, uses trigger points
  - Isometric contraction – contraction without joint movement
  - Isotonic contraction – contraction with joint movement
  - Isokinetic contraction – movement at a constant speed through a range of motion with mild resistance

Stretching:
- Assisted static stretching – therapists assists client in stretching until resistance is met
- Unassisted static stretching – client stretches into resistance and applies light contraction, such as in yoga
- Ballistic stretching - bobbing or bouncing during the stretch, not recommended due to possibility of muscle strain or tear
- Passive stretching – slow gentle movement to lengthen muscles when resistance is minimal

End feel - change in quality of movement at first sign of resistance:
- Normal end feel – limit on range of motion of a joint
- Hard end feel – bone against bone
- Soft end feel – cushioned limitation
- Empty end feel – abrupt restriction to joint movement

Joint movements:
- Active – client participates
- Passive – client remain relaxed

If a client is functioning from sympathetic nervous system dominance, an appropriate initial stroke would be tapotement.
If a client is functioning from parasympathetic nervous system dominance, an appropriate initial stroke would be gentle rocking.

E. Hot / Cold Applications

Hydrotherapy – hot or cold massage application using hot or cold water
Thermotherapy - external application of heat for therapeutic purposes

Contrast method:
- Hydrotherapy application that combines heat and cold
- Benefits include alternating vasoconstriction and vasodilatation
- Beneficial for chronic muscle spasms

Cryotherapy - the external application of cold for therapeutic purposes
    including ice massage

Slight analgesia - neurological state in which painful stimuli are
    moderated

R.I.C.E.S. First Aid principle – Rest, Ice, Compression, Elevation,
    Stabilization, appropriate for sprains and strains

Hydrotherapy applications:
- Fomentations - hot packs
- Pack - a bag or sack used to apply heat or cold
- Compress - a wet cloth with water wrung from it that is applied to
  the skin's surface
- Infrared radiation produced from bulb or element
- Friction rubs - body polishes, cold mittens, dry brush massages,
  ice massages, salt glows, and shampoos
- Sauna - uses hot air from 170 to 210 degrees Fahrenheit with 10%
  to 20% humidity
- Salt rub - friction with a saline solution
- Sponging - hydrotherapy applications using friction
- Diathermy – application of oscillating magnetic fields to tissue

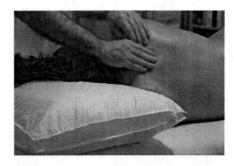

Baths:

- Bath - broad category of hydrotherapy application that involves partial or complete immersion in water
- Steam bath - uses hot vapors in a confined area for temperatures from 105 to 120 degrees Fahrenheit with 100% humidity
- Shower or spray - streams of water under pressure
- Immersion bath - the client sitting in a tub
- Whirlpool - the client sitting in a tub and receiving jets of water against the skin
- Sitz bath (hip bath) - a sitting bath with the water coming up to the navel
- Saline bath - a bath with salt
- Body shampoo - scrubbing the body with a brush dipped in warm, soapy water
- Russian bath – full-body steam bath

Effects of Heat

Increased blood flow
Increased metabolism
Reduced pain
Increased range of motion
Decreased stiffness

Effects of Cold and Ice

Reduced inflammation
Reduced swelling (antiedemic)
Reduced muscle spasm
Vasoconstriction initially induced
Secondary effect of increased local circulation
Initial feeling of uncomfortable cold
Eventual feeling of total numbness

Conditions for which heat could be applied:

- Impaired circulation
- Arthritis
- Increasing extensibility of collagen tissue

Conditions for which cold could be applied:
- Swelling, reducing spasticity
- Prevent injury to tissue

Application of ice:
- Ice pack
- Ice in a plastic bag
- Ice wrapped in towel
- Ice in paper or Styrofoam cup

Avoid hydrotherapy:
- Extremely high or low blood pressure
- Lung disease
- Cardiac impairment
- Infectious skin condition
- Diabetes
- Kidney infection

Avoid ice and cold:
- Circulatory problems
- Cold applications not used for prolonged periods because of depressing effects

Avoid heat:
- Inflammation
- Edema
- Acute stage of injury

Temperatures:
- Temperature of a warm bath - 95 to 100 degrees Fahrenheit or 35 to 38 degrees Celsius
- Temperature of a hot bath - 100 to 110 degrees Fahrenheit or 38 to 43 degrees Celsius
- Temperature of water that can cause tissue damage - below 30 degrees Fahrenheit or above 124 degrees Fahrenheit, below 0 degrees Celsius or above 51 degrees Celsius
- Neutral water temperature - 92 to 93 degrees Fahrenheit or 32 to 33 degrees Celsius
- Maximum temperature that the skin can tolerate for a hot bath - 115 degrees Fahrenheit or 46 degrees Celsius
- Maximum temperature that the skin can tolerate for steam vapor - 140 degrees Fahrenheit or 60 degrees Celsius
- Water temperature that after a prolonged period would raise the body temperature to a dangerous level - 110 degrees Fahrenheit or 43 degrees Celsius

V. Client Assessment, Reassessment & Treatment Planning

A. Organization of a Massage / Bodywork Session

Massage Session:
1. Appointment
2. Intake and Medical History forms
3. Consultation
4. Perform massage
5. Update SOAP chart and client records

Intake and medical history forms – information for the therapist to use to develop treatment strategy, health history and contact information

Pain questionnaire – scale for communicating level of discomfort

Care plan - client goals and a time frame

If a client only has 30 minutes for a massage instead of the usual hour, the duration would be adjusted.

Positions:
- Prone position - lying face down
- Supine position - lying face up, more comfortable position for clients with allergies and cold-related respiratory congestion
- Side-lying or laterally recumbent position - lying on the side, good position to start a massage for a pregnant client
- Erect position - standing up
- Seated position – in a chair, good position for the client when performing on-site corporate massage

Prone position:
- Good position to start a massage for first-time clients to make them feel more comfortable and safer
- Good position to start a massage for clients with back pain and tension
- Good position massaging the biceps femoris

The best way to turn a client is to hold the edge of the sheet and have the client turn towards therapist.

Self care recommendations - suggestions that support the client in achieving their goals
Self help - recommendation for activities between sessions
Treatment plan - recommendations for future treatment

In general, about one or two stretches should be recommended for homework.

B. Client Consultation and Evaluation

The Consultation:
1. Greet client
2. Determine client's needs
3. Explain procedures
4. State policies
5. Perform preliminary assessment
6. Formulate treatment plan
7. Obtain informed consent from client

If a client says an area is stiff, it is usually a connective tissue or fluid retention issue.
If a client says an area is tight, it is usually a muscle tone issue.
If a client says an area is stuck, it is usually a joint issue.

Diminished blood flow could cause a cold area.
A muscle spasm could cause a hot area.

Target muscle - the muscle being treated in a therapeutic technique
Tense muscle - too strong

Identify concentrically contracted shortened areas so that correction can be applied to those areas.
The appropriate massage technique for shortened muscles is to lengthen and stretch.
After identifying short tissues, lengthen and stretch tight areas
Massage methods usually produce longer muscles.
Massaging tight but long functioning muscle areas could add to muscle imbalance.

A client who had recently ruptured an Achilles tendon would most likely have spasms and pain in the gastrocnemius and soleus muscles.

C. Written Data Collection

SOAP Headings

Subjective
Objective
Assessment
Plan

Subjective:
- List of prioritized health concerns or goals for the session
- Verbal information that clients share (client says they did not sleep well, client describes pain)
- Activities that aggravate or relieve the symptoms
- Written information that clients share regarding health history
- Symptoms related to the current health concerns

Objective:
- Therapist's visual observations, such as observation of muscle guarding
- Palpation findings
- Initial gait analysis
- Massage treatment applications including techniques, duration, and location
- Patient's response to the massage (could also be considered assessment)
- Range-of-motion testing
- Physical assessment

Assessment:
- Short-term goals based on the activities of daily living recorded
- Long-term goals
- Functional outcomes
- Massage treatment given
- Changes due to massage
- Progress related to session

Plan:
- Test recommendations
- Self care recommendations, such as stretches
- Referrals
- Functional outcomes

SOAPIER headings:
- Subjective
- Objective
- Assessment
- Plan
- Intervention
- Evaluation
- Revisions

D. Visual Assessment

Gait assessment	observing basic body movements of walking to recognize dysfunctional and inefficient patterns
Posture assessment	observing the client's gravitation line, balance and symmetry in various positions
Functional assessment	the efficiency of coordinated movement
Needs assessment	more of a part of developing a plan than an objective observation

Effects of Gravity:
- Coronal plane - the gravity line in the side view of standing posture
- Midsagittal plane - the gravity line in the back view of standing posture
- The body must be balanced in all three dimensions to withstand the forces of gravity
- With ideally aligned posture, the center of gravity is slightly anterior to the first or second sacral segment
- The atlas is an area where the body is balanced in gravity
- The flexor and adductor muscles usually work against gravity

Postural Analysis

Ideal alignment in the posterior view:
- Level shoulders
- Medial borders of scapulae parallel
- Feet parallel or slight out-toeing
- Level pelvis
- Straight spine

Lordotic Posture

Lordosis, hyperextended lumbar spine, anterior tilt of the pelvis
Low back muscles most likely short and strong
Anterior abdominals elongated and weak
Hamstrings somewhat elongated and may or may not be weak
Hip flexors short and strong

Kyphotic-Lordotic Posture

Kyphosis and Lordosis, including forward head
Hamstrings slightly elongated but may or may not be weak
Upper back erector spinae elongated and weak
Neck flexors elongated and weak
External obliques elongated and weak
Neck extensors short and strong
Low back muscles are strong and may or may not develop shortness
Hip flexors short and strong

Flat back posture:
- Flexed or straight lumbar spine
- Forward head
- Flexed or straight lumbar spine
- Posterior pelvic tilt
- One-joint hip flexors elongated and weak
- Hamstrings short and strong

Sway-back posture:
- Forward head
- Increased flexion in thoracic spine
- Posterior pelvic tilt
- One-joint hip flexors elongated and weak
- Upper fibers of the internal obliques short and strong
- Hamstrings short and strong
- External obliques and upper back extensors elongated and weak
- One-joint hip flexors elongated and weak
- Neck flexors elongated and weak

Forward Head Position

Short and strong neck extensors
Long and weak anterior vertebral neck flexors
The neck rotators are long

Forward head and round upper back:
- Tension headaches
- Tight muscles in the back of the neck

Scapulae in good alignment:
- Flat against the upper back about 4 inches apart
- Medial borders of scapulae parallel

Neutral position of the pelvis:
- Pelvis in ideal alignment
- Normal anterior curve of the low back
- The abdominal muscles pull upward
- The posterior hip flexors pull downward
- The back muscles pull upward
- The anterior hip flexors pull downward

Faulty posture of the pelvis:
- Posterior pelvic tilt – sway-back or flat back
- Weak abdominal muscles would most likely allow the pelvis to tilt forward
- Anterior pelvic tilt – lordotic posture

Good alignment of the knees:
- The patella face forward
- The plumb line passes slightly anterior to the axis of the knee joint
- Standard side-view line of reference through the lower extremities passes posterior to the center of the hip joint and anterior to the axis of the knee joint

Faulty posture of the knees:
- Genu varum – bowlegs (<>)
- Genu valgum - knock-knees (><)
- When knees are in hyperextension, the ankle joint is in plantar flexion

Good alignment of the feet:
- The feet are not in pronation
- The feet are not in supination
- Slight out-toeing
- Heels 3 inches apart and angle of out-toeing 8 to 10 degrees from the midline
- Standard side-view line of reference through the ankle passes anterior to the outer malleolus and through the apex of the arch

Faulty posture of the feet:
- Flat foot - low longitudinal arch
- Calluses under ball of foot - low metatarsal arch
- Pronation - ankle rolls in
- Supination - ankle rolls out
- Pigeon-toed - the toes are in while walking
- Slue-footed - the toes are out while walking

Shoes with heels:
- In-toeing or pigeon-toes increase with heel height
- Tendency toward parallel position from out-toeing increases with heel height
- Gastrocnemius and soleus are shortened by wearing high heeled shoes

The plumb line is used as a reference when viewing a standing posture.

If posture is not balanced, postural muscles must function more like ligaments and bones.

Ergonomic Factors

Ergonomics - coordinates activities with work equipment

Correct set up for proper ergonomics at a computer workstation:
- Monitor at or below eye level
- Phone headset
- Chair has armrests

Incorrect set up considering ergonomics at a computer workstation:
- Computer in a corner on a platform
- Phone on shoulder
- Feet propped on chair legs
- Computer in a corner on a platform

Good alignment for sitting posture:
- The position requires the least expenditure of muscle energy
- 90 degree angle for the hip and knees for good alignment in sitting posture
- 10 degree incline for the back of a chair for good alignment in sitting posture

Armrests of a chair:
- When the armrests of a chair are too high, the shoulders will be pushed upward
- When the armrests of a chair are too low, the arms will not have proper support

Proprioception of Movement

Walking:
- When standing in heels or walking fast, the feet tend to become parallel
- Walking with lateral rotation of the legs puts strain on the longitudinal arches

When the foot speed increases from walking to sprinting:
- The heels do not contact the ground
- The weight is borne on the anterior side of the foot
- There is a tendency for in-toeing

Protective muscle contraction could be the result of inefficient joint movement during walking that could lead to tissue shortening.

E. Palpation Assessment

Palpation:
- The use of touch to examine tissues
- Used to find tender areas within muscles resulting from a postural deviation
- Temperature, texture, tenderness and tone

Tender point - a small painful area of hypertonicity

Bony landmarks that are processes to which tendons and ligaments attach:
- Crest, epicondyle, line, spine, trochanter, tuberosity
- Lamina groove - progresses down the spine
- Olecranon process - the bony landmark used to locate the proximal end of the ulna
- Carotid tubercle - found near C-6
- Jugular notch, sternal angle, and xiphoid process - located at T2, T4 and T10 of the vertebral column

Trigger points - Refer symptoms to other areas of the body

Brachial plexus impingement - trigger points along the lateral neck flexors, horizontal arm abductors, internal arm rotators
Low back pain - trigger points along the psoas, quadratus lumborum, and hamstrings

Referred pain:
- Trigger point on the deltoid – refers pain down the lateral side of the arm
- Trigger point on the sternocleidomastoid - refers pain to the head and face, occipital regions, ear, forehead
- Trigger point on the piriformis - refers pain to the sacroiliac region, buttock and down posterior thigh
- Trigger point on tensor fasciae latae - refers pain to the hip and down lateral side of leg
- Trigger point on latissimus dorsi - refers pain to the posterior axillary area, scapula, and ulnar side of arm
- Trigger point on orbicularis oculi - refers pain above eyelid, sinuses

Pressure on a trigger point typically must be maintained for 30 to 45 seconds until the tissue releases.

Muscle guarding - involves a hypertonic muscle stabilizing or splinting an area

Character armor - the concept that the suppression of emotions causes muscular tension

F. Range of Motion Assessment

Normal end feel - the limit on the range of motion of a joint

Abnormal end feel - what occurs when there is no physical restriction to movement other than the pain expressed by the client

Anatomic position is zero (0) degrees of motion.

When the range of motion of a joint allows 0 to 90 degrees of flexion, anything less is hypomobile.

When the range of motion of a joint allows 0 to 90 degrees of flexion, anything more is hypermobile.

When assessing the function of the shoulder, resistance is applied at the distal end of the humerus.

When assessing extension of the hip, resistance is applied at the end of the femur.

When assessing flexion of the knee, resistance is applied at the distal end of the tibia.

Joint Movement Techniques

Decreased range of motion in horizontal abduction and lateral rotation of the shoulder:
Lengthen upper fibers of pectoralis major

Decreased overhead range of motion in flexion and abduction of the shoulder:
Lengthen lower fibers of pectoralis major

Arm pain and a depressed coracoid process of the scapula:
Lengthen pectoralis minor

Achilles tendinitis and pain behind the knee when flexing the knee:
* Hamstrings are weak
* Gastrocnemius is overactive

Limited range of motion in lateral rotation and abduction of the shoulder:
Lengthen teres major

Plantar tendinitis and knee pain under the patella when extending knee:
- Vastus lateralis is overactive
- Vastus medius is weak

Low back pain, buttock pain, and hamstring shortening when flexing the trunk:
- Erector spinae, psoas, and rectus abdominis are overactive
- Abdominal complex muscles are weak

Low back pain, buttock pain, and hamstring strains when extending the trunk:
- Erector spinae and hamstrings are overactive
- Gluteus maximum is weak

Shoulder pain, low back pain, and a headache when flexing the shoulders:
- Upper trapezius and ipsilateral quadratus lumborum are overactive
- Levator scapula is weak

Structural and Functional Integration

Testing the arms:
- Test the left arm flexors - client holds left arm position against therapist's inferior/caudal pressure
- Test the left arm extensors - client holds left arm position against therapist's superior/cephalad pressure
- Test the right arm extensors - client holds right arm position against therapist's superior/cephalad pressure
- Test the right arm flexors - client holds right arm position against therapist's inferior/caudal pressure
- Test the arm adductors - client holds position against therapist's lateral pressure on arms

Testing the legs:
- Test the left leg flexors - client holds left leg position against therapist's inferior/caudal pressure
- Test the left leg extensors - client holds left leg position against therapist's superior/cephalad pressure
- Test the right leg extensors - client holds right leg position against therapist's superior/cephalad pressure
- Test the right leg flexors - client holds right leg position against therapist's inferior/caudal pressure
- Test the leg adductors - client holds position against therapist's lateral pressure on legs

To work on a client's serratus anterior, adduct the arm.

Stretch the pectoralis major for kyphosis.

Put a pillow under the abducted bent elbow, with client in supine position, to work on a client's pectoralis minor.

If an athlete complains of pain in the patella after an event, massage the quadriceps.

The sternocleidomastoid (SCM) muscle is associated with spasmodic torticollis.

To stretch the pectoralis major, abduct and laterally rotate the arm.

G. Clinical Reasoning

Tendinitis:
- Inflammation of a tendon due to overuse
- Heat and swelling may be palpated at tendon
- Painful around tendon
- Apply cold in acute stage to reduce inflammation
- Apply heat in chronic stage to soften adhesions and increase circulation
- Stretch shortened muscles
- Strengthen weak muscles
- Reduce pain
- Reduce hypertonicity and trigger points
- Mobilize hypomobile joints

Rotator cuff tendinitis - may be caused by throwing sports such as baseball or occupations such as drywall hanging

Tennis elbow:
- Lateral epicondylitis
- Inflammation of the common extensor tendon
- Can be caused by occupations such as plumbing and meat cutting

Golfer's elbow:
- Medial epicondylitis
- Inflammation of the common flexor tendon
- Can be caused by occupations requiring hammering or using a screwdriver

Thoracic Outlet Syndrome

Nerve compression syndrome
Condition that involves compression of the brachial plexus and artery
Lengthen scalenes, SCMs, pecs, and neck extensors

Anterior scalene syndrome – between anterior and middle scalene
Pectoralis minor syndrome – between coracoids process and pec minor
Costoclavicular syndrome – between clavicle and first rib

Trigger finger – swelling of tendons in finger due to overuse

Bursitis
- Inflammation of a bursa caused by overuse of structures surrounding the bursa
- Bursa – small fluid-filled sac that reduces friction
- Baker's cyst – synovial cyst that usually appears on lateral side of popliteal space
- Bunion – excessive bone growth at first metatarsophalangeal joint capsule
- Avoid compressing the bursa
- Swelling and redness can be observed over more superficial bursa and heat is palpated locally
- Apply cold in acute stage and deep moist heat in chronic stage
- Friction may be applied to area surrounding the bursa
- Joint play is indicated for hypomobile joints

Shoulders and Scapulae

Upper trapezius tight when the shoulders are elevated and the scapulae adducted
Upper trapezius weak when the shoulders are depressed and the scapulae abducted
Upper trapezius needs to be exercised when the shoulders are depressed and the scapulae abducted
Serratus anterior and trapezius are weak when the scapula is rotated so the axillary border is more horizontal than normal
Serratus anterior is weak when the scapula is rotated so the axillary border is more horizontal than normal

Frozen shoulder
- Painful significant restriction of active and passive range of motion at the shoulder
- Most frequently in abduction and external rotation

Causes of frozen shoulder:
- Intrinsic musculoskeletal trauma
- Trigger points in subscapularis
- Could be caused by hyperkyphosis

Stages of frozen shoulder:
- Acute – freezing phase or first stage
- Subacute – frozen phase or second stage
- Chronic – thawing phase or third stage

Treatment of frozen shoulder
- Ice in acute stage and heat in subacute and chronic stages
- treat compensating structures
- mobilize hypomobile joints
- reduce fascial restrictions
- increase range of motion
- reduce hypertonicity and trigger points

Tight muscles from holding a telephone on the right shoulder:
Lengthen right upper trapezius

Tight muscles from holding a telephone on the left shoulder:
Lengthen left splenius

Retracted shoulders:
Stretch rhomboids

Adducted and elevated scapula:
Lengthen trapezius

Head and neck

Torticollis:
- Abnormal positioning of the head and neck relative to the body
- Treat and stretch affected sternocleidomastoid muscle
- Acute acquired torticollis – painful unilateral shortening or spasm of neck muscles resulting in an abnormal head position
- Congenital torticollis – contracture of one sternocleidomastoid muscle resulting in an abnormal head position

Left torticollis:
Lengthen left splenius capitis and right upper trapezius

Right torticollis:
Lengthen right splenius capitis and left upper trapezius

Forward head position:
- Lengthen and stretch cervical spine extensors
- Lengthen and stretch levator
- Lengthen and stretch upper trapezius

Whiplash:
- Acceleration/deceleration injury to the head and neck
- Forward head posture
- Increase in cervical lordotic curve
- Reduce hypertonicity and trigger points in neck and shoulders
- Treat SCM trigger points
- Reduce hypertonicity and trigger points in infra- and supra-hyoid muscles
- Gradually increase range of motion

Postural Balancing - Spine

Flat-back posture:
- Posterior pelvic tilt and hip extension
- Stretch tight hamstrings and abdominals
- Lengthen biceps femoris
- Lengthen semitendinosus

Hyperlordosis:
- Increase in normal lumbar lordotic curve
- Increased anterior pelvic tilt and hip flexion
- Sway-back posture
- Lengthen tight iliopsoas, rectus femoris, tensor fascia lata, and adductors
- Lengthen tight erector spinae and quadrates lumborum
- Gluteus maximus and hamstrings are weak
- Abdominals are weak

Hyperkyphosis:
- Increase in normal thoracic kyphotic curve
- Protracted scapulae and head-forward posture
- Lengthen tight pecs, subclavius, serratus anterior, and anterior intercostals
- Lengthen tight SCM, upper trapezius, suboccipitals, levator scapulae, and scalene
- Rhomboids, middle trapezius, thoracic erector spinae, supra-hyoids, infra-hyoids, longus capitis, and longus cervicis are weak
- May accompany flat-back posture
- May have accompanying hyperlordosis

Kyphotic-Lordotic Posture

Lengthen iliacus and rectus capitis posterior major
Lengthen psoas major and upper trapezius
Lengthen rectus femoris and splenius
Lengthen adductor longus and oblique capitis superior

Lordotic Posture

Lengthen tensor fasciae latae and longissimus thoracis
Lengthen rectus femoris and quadratus lumborum
Lengthen psoas major and multifidi
Stretch low back muscles
Lengthen iliacus and iliocostalis lumborum

Scoliosis:
- Lateral rotary deviation of the spine
- Traditionally C-curve or S-curve
- Lengthen the short latissimus dorsi

C-curve of the back:
Lengthen short lateral internal and external obliques

Rotation of the thorax forward on the left:
Lengthen left internal and right external obliques

Tendency towards kyphosis and a depressed chest:

Lengthen anterior internal and external obliques

Knees, legs, and hips

Piriformis syndrome:
- Compression of the sciatic nerve by the piriformis muscle
- Refers pain down posterior thigh
- Treat by reducing compression on sciatic nerve

Patellofemoral syndrome:
- Painful degenerative changes to articular cartilage on the underside of the patella
- Treat IT band, hamstrings, adductors and, quadriceps

Iliotibial band contracture:
- Contracture or thickening of the iliotibial (IT) band
- Focus treatment on IT band
- IT band is muscle that provides lateral support at the knee
- Stretch tensor fascia lata and gluteus maximus

Prominent or high right hip:
- Stretch right lateral trunk muscles
- Stretch left lateral thigh muscles

Prominent or high left hip:
- Stretch left lateral trunk muscles
- Stretch right lateral thigh muscles

Toeing out when walking:
Stretch the plantar flexor muscles

Flexed knee:
- Stretch knee flexors and hip flexors
- Stretch hip medial rotators

Knock-knees:
Stretch the fascia lata

Hammer toes and a low metatarsal arch:
Stretch the metatarsophalangeal joints

Right hip adducted and medially rotated, left hip abducted and feet in pronation:
- Short and strong right lateral trunk muscles, right hip adductors and left hip abductors
- Short and strong left peroneus longus and brevis and right tibialis posterior
- Short and strong right flexor hallucis longus and right flexor digitorum longus
- Long and weak left lateral trunk muscles, right hip abductors and left hip adductors
- Long and weak right peroneus longus and brevis and left tibialis posterior
- Long and weak left flexor hallucis longus and left flexor digitorum longus

Left hip adducted and medially rotated, right hip abducted and feet in pronation:
- Short and strong left lateral trunk muscles, right hip abductors and left hip adductors
- Short and strong right peroneus longus and brevis and left tibialis posterior
- Short and strong left flexor hallucis longus and left flexor digitorum longus
- Long and weak right lateral trunk muscles, left hip abductors and right hip adductors
- Long and weak left peroneus longus and brevis and right tibialis posterior
- Long and weak right flexor hallucis longus and right flexor digitorum longus

Medially rotated femur:
Stretch the hip medial rotators

Hyperextended knees when standing and the toes out when walking:
Lengthen soleus

Knee in a flexed position with medial rotation of the leg on the thigh:
Lengthen popliteus

Knee flexed along with posterior tilting of the pelvis and a flattening of the lumbar spine:
Lengthen hamstrings

Restricted flexion of the knee:
Lengthen quadriceps femoris

Flexion, abduction, and lateral rotation deformity of the hip, with flexion of the knee:
Lengthen sartorius

Hip in a flexed position and a knock-knee position:
Lengthen tensor fasciae latae

Thigh in a position of abduction and medial rotation, with a lateral pelvic tilt:
Lengthen gluteus minimus

Abduction deformity that may be seen as a lateral pelvic tilt:
Lengthen gluteus medius

The adductors, tensor fasciae latae, and quadratus lumborum muscles are overactive if a client has pain in the low back, buttocks, sacroiliac joint, lateral knee, and anterior knee.

The gluteus medius muscle is weak if a client has pain in the low back, buttocks, sacroiliac joint, lateral knee, and anterior knee.

Feet

Plantar fasciitis:
- Overuse condition resulting in an inflammation of the plantar fascia
- Plantar fascia attaches to calcaneus and merges to plantar joints
- Pain is worse during toe-off stage of gait
- Palpation of calcaneus is painful
- Apply cold in acute stage
- Apply deep moist heat in chronic stage
- Treat the shortened gastrocnemius and soleus
- Thumb kneading on plantar surface of foot
- Cross fiber friction on adhesions in plantar fascia

Client walks with the toes out:
Stretch plantar flexors

Foot pulled into forefoot varus with the big toe abducted:
Lengthen abductor hallucis

Hallux valgus (bunion deformity):
Lengthen adductor hallucis

Extended great toe, with the head of the first metatarsal driven
   downward:
Lengthen extensor hallucis longus

Flexion deformity of the distal phalanges of the lateral four toes:
Lengthen flexor digitorum longus

Dorsiflexion of the ankle joint, with inversion of the foot:
Lengthen tibialis anterior

Supinated position of the heel with forefoot varus:
Lengthen tibialis posterior

Everted or valgus position of the foot:
Lengthen peroneus brevis

Arms and wrists

Carpal tunnel syndrome:
   • Most common entrapment syndrome in arm
   • Condition that results from the compression of the median nerve
     as it passes through the carpal tunnel at the wrist
   • Results in numbing and tingling in the lateral three and one-half
     digits
   • Treat pronator teres and muscles that pass through carpal tunnel
   • Decrease compression on median nerve

Wrist flexed to the radial side:
Lengthen flexor carpi radialis

Wrist flexed to the ulnar side:
Lengthen flexor carpi ulnaris

Coracoid process depressed anteriorly when the arm is at the side:
Lengthen coracobrachialis

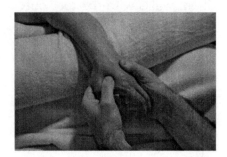

Right handed / left handed individuals

Muscles that tend to show acquired postural weakness in right handed individuals:
- Right hip abductors
- Right hip lateral rotators
- Right peroneus longus and brevis
- Left flexor digitorum longus
- Left flexor hallucis longus
- Left tibialis anterior
- Left lateral trunk muscles

Muscles that tend to show acquired postural weakness in left handed individuals:
- Left hip abductors
- Left hip lateral rotators
- Left peroneus longus and brevis
- Right flexor digitorum longus
- Right flexor hallucis longus
- Right tibialis anterior
- Right lateral trunk muscles

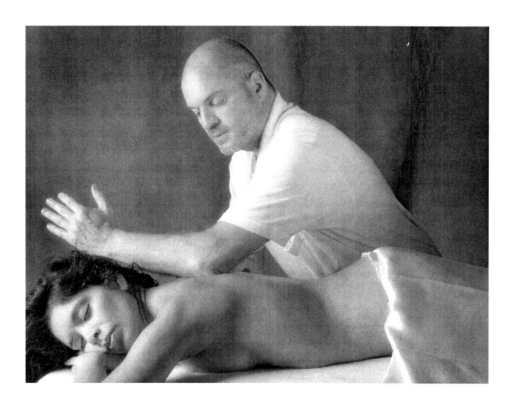

VI. Overview of Massage & Bodywork History / Culture / Modalities

A. History of Massage and Bodywork

Per Henrik Ling	developed Swedish massage, the father of Swedish massage and physical therapy, called system of movements medical gymnastics
John Grosvenor	English surgeon who practiced chirurgy, healing with the hands
Dr. Johann Georg Mezger	standardized massage terminology and is given credit for bringing massage to the scientific community
Dr. George H. Taylor	popularized the Movement Cure in America, introducing the Swedish movements in the mid 19th century
Elizabeth Dicke	developed connective tissue massage or Bindegewebmassage, a structural and postural integration approach, because she was suffering from impaired circulation in the leg
Dr. Emil Vodder and Dr. Estrid Vodder	developed manual lymph drainage, a light massage technique
James Cyriax	developed deep transverse friction, soft tissue manipulation
Boris Chaitow and Stanley Leif	developed neuromuscular therapy, a soft tissue method
Dr. William Fitzgerald and Eunice Ingram	developed reflexology based on Asian roots
Paul St. John	developed neuromuscular approach, a nervous or reflexive method
Janet Travel	Developed procedure based on trigger points
Joseph Heller	developed Hellerwork, a structural integration approach
John F. Barnes	formalized myofascial approach focusing on connective tissue
Randolph Stone	Developed polarity theory
Dr. Milton Trager	Developed the Trager method
Dr. Ida Rolf	Developed Rolfing©
Dr. John Thie	Developed Touch for Health
Dr. John Upledger	Developed craniosacral therapy

Chinese anmo techniques:
- Earliest massage techniques including rubbing, pressing, and manipulations
- Acupressure stems from acupuncture
- Stimulation of acupuncture points to regulate chi, the life force energy

Japanese massage:
- Shiatsu - a Japanese massage technique comes from a word for finger pressure
- Tsubo – points sensitive to pressure applied during Shiatsu
- Amma - traditional Japanese massage technique comes from a Chinese word for calming by rubbing

Indian and Hindu massage:
- Ayurveda - developed in India
- Tschanpua – Hindu technique of massage in the bath

Greek massage:
- Gymnasium – center for exercise and massage
- Ascete – person who exercises mind and body
- Hippocratic Oath – code of ethics for physicians
- Anatripsis – art of rubbing a body part upward

Swedish system:
- Based on Western concepts of anatomy and physiology
- Employs traditional manipulative techniques
  - Effleurage
  - Petrissage
  - Vibration
  - Friction
  - Tapotement

German method:
- Combines many of the Swedish movements
- Emphasizes the use of various therapeutic baths

French and English systems – also employ many of the Swedish massage movements

Massage Theory

Intuition - knowing something without going through a conscious process of thinking

Art - a craft, skill, technique, or talent

Science - the intellectual process of using all resources available to better understand and predict natural phenomena

The hypothesis is tested through experiments.

Research is validated with further research to replicate findings.

The National Institute of Health Office of Alternative and Complementary Medicine is an organization primarily focused on research.

B. Overview of the Different Skill Sets used in Contemporary Massage / Bodywork Environments

Manual lymphatic drainage - best for removing waste

Trigger point therapy:
- Best for tight bands of muscle fibers
- Identifies tender spots on muscle tissues that can refer pain to other parts of the body

Neuromuscular therapy (NMT):
- Relieves tender muscle tissue and compressed nerves that refer pain
- Focuses on pain and explores the soft tissue components of pain
- Gliding – primary technique of NMT uses the thumb across tissues
- Ischemic compression – digital pressure directly on a trigger point
  - Duration of pressure 8 to 12 seconds
- Skin rolling – a variation of kneading
- Stretching – passive and active stretching of muscle and connective tissue

Sports Massage:
- Rehabilitation massage - used for severe injuries
- Recovery massage - given after an event when there are no injuries present
- Remedial massage - used for minor injuries
- Active joint movements - effective for flexibility during sports massage

Reflexology:
- Applies pressure to points on the hands and feet
- Diaphragm line - across the ball of the foot
- Waist line -across the metatarsals
- Heel line -across the calcaneus
- Brain - reflex point is associated with the great toe
- Heart - reflex point is proximal to the great toe and medial to the ball of the foot
- Shoulder - reflex point is proximal to the great toe and lateral to the ball of the foot
- Sinuses - reflex point is associated with the four lateral toes
- Stomach - reflex point is on the medial side of the foot in between the waist line and diaphragm line

Feldenkrais therapy - change movement patterns and improves posture

Ortho-bionomy -a non-invasive neuromuscular approach with roots in osteopathy

Craniosacral therapy - manipulating the rhythmic flow of the cerebrospinal fluid, uses the principles of unwinding

Lomi lomi – Hawaiian manipulative massage technique

Esalen massage:
- Developed in California
- Uses long flowing strokes that connect all parts of the body into a whole

Complementary bodywork systems:
- Hydrotherapy
- Lymphatic drainage
- Reflexology
- Connective tissue approaches
- Trigger point therapy
- Asian bodywork methods
- Ayurveda
- Polarity therapy

Professionals providing opportunities for massage therapists:
- Chiropractors
- Physicians
- Physical therapists

C. Overview of Massage / Bodywork Modalities

Classifications of touch technique:
Mechanical or expressive touch

Static Touch / Holding

Grounding - establishes a boundary between the therapist and the client

Energetic effects of massage:
- Improving the flow of energy within or around the body
- Biofields or energetic methods
- Healing energy and the subtle energy fields around the body

Energy techniques:
- Therapeutic Touch - non-invasive touch
- Reiki – energy technique without direct touching
- Touch for Health
- Polarity Therapy

Polarity Therapy:
- Primary goal of releasing energy
- Based on a balance flow of energy as an important element for a healthy body
- Right side - positive expanding energy
- Left side - negative receptive energy
- Five major body currents -ether, air, fire, water, and earth
- Reflexes - points along an energy current that connect with other points along that current
- Blocked Energy - what polarity therapy attempts to locate and release

Aromatherapy:
- Aromatherapy - use of scented oils and lotions to stimulate olfactory nerve
- Relaxing - lavender, clary sage, melissa, ylang ylang, bergamot and chamomile
- Stimulating - rosemary, thyme, pine and cypress
- Soothing - chamomile, jasmine, geranium, and rose
- Moisturizing - orange blossom, neroli, patchouli and lavender

Overview of Energy Modalities

Meridians or channels - an energy flow along a nerve tract

Chi or Qi or Ki - a life force or energy

Tao - the path or way to sustain energy
Acupressure - based on about 360 points of energy
Tsubos - reactive points in Shiatsu, acupressure, and acupuncture

Yang - the light, energetic aspect of the universe
Yin - the dark, dense, deep aspect of the universe

Governing Vessel - responsible for all yang meridians
Conception Vessel - responsible for all yin meridians

Shiatsu:
- Kata - a sequence of movements
- Jitsu - an area of excessively strong ki
- Kyo - an area of deficient and weak ki
- Japanese massage

Ayurveda:
- Doshas - energy forces
    o Kapha - associated with mucus
    o Vata - associated with the wind
    o Pitta - associated with bile
- Indian and Hindu massage

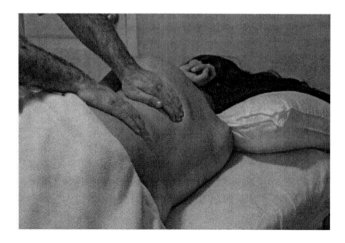

VII. Ethics, Boundaries, Laws, Regulations

A. Ethical Behavior

Code of ethics - commonly accepted guidelines or principles of conduct that govern professional conduct, guidelines for morally acceptable and professional behavior

Ethics - guiding principles for distinguishing between right and wrong

Associated Bodywork & Massage Professionals (ABMP) Code of Ethics:
- Client Relationships
- Professionalism
- Scope of Practice / Appropriate Techniques
- Image / Advertising Claims

NCBTMB Standards of Practice:
- Prevention of sexual misconduct - contains guidelines for sexual conduct and guidance on breast massage
- Confidentiality - guidance on client files and sharing information
- Business practices - guidance on insurance and accounting
- Professionalism - guidance on hygiene and draping, guidance on peer review and the scope of practice
- Legal and Ethical Requirements - guidance on violations and complaints
- Roles and boundaries - guidance on personal limitations and relationships
- Business practices - guidance on advertising and fees

If a minor asks the therapist to make an exception and give a massage without permission from a parent or legal guardian, the therapist should not give the massage.

If a client reveals that they are guilty of child abuse, the law may require that the client be reported to child welfare authorities.

Duties:
Do no harm
Do positive good

The "Do no harm" duty is more compelling than the "Do positive good" duty if the two are in conflict.

B. Professional Boundaries

Boundary – like a protective circle around the professional relationship that separates what is appropriate from what is not
Boundaries – Lines that separate, limits, barriers, borders, and edges
Types of Boundaries – interpersonal, emotional, sexual, and intellectual
How to create, manage, and change boundaries – power differences, time, location, language, clothing, space, touch, money, dual relationships, self-disclosure

Contract – an agreement between practitioner and client that is often implied rather than explicit about what each will or will not do
Client-centered – actions and words motivated by what is best for the client

Transference:
- When a client's expectations and behaviors are moved to the therapist
- A client's feelings towards the therapist
- Often based on fantasy or feelings towards another person in the past
- For example, the client gives the therapists gifts that show affection

Countertransference:
- When a therapist's expectations and behaviors are moved to the client
- The feelings of a therapist towards the client
- The response of the therapist's unconscious toward the client
- For example, when a therapist gets angry because the client is talking too much or complaining about personal problems

Projection – when a person has uncomfortable feelings and projects them onto others

If a practitioner is sad or angry, then the practitioner is projecting by making the assumption that a client is sad or angry.

If a client does not want to fill out a medical history form, the client may feel that the disclosure would cross a boundary and the therapist should offer alternatives such as taking the information verbally or filling out a shorter form.

If a therapist takes on symptoms and conditions experienced by clients, the therapist may has an excessively permeable boundary.

85

If a therapist for the first time suddenly gives a regular client a big hug after the session, the therapist has crossed the client's boundary.

If a client leaves underwear on and the therapist removes underwear or unsnaps a bra without asking for permission, the therapist has violated the client's boundaries.

C. Code of Ethics Violations

Examples of Violations of Codes of Ethics:
- Practicing beyond scope of practice – spinal adjustments, massage or counseling without proper training
- Sexual misconduct – watching a client undress or hugging a client in a sexual way
- Misrepresentation of educational status – implying that attending a workshop is the same as an advanced degree
- Financial impropriety – changing different fees for cash-paying clients and clients with insurance
- Exploiting the power differential – asking a professional for advice during the treatment
- Misleading claims of creative abilities – guaranteeing that pain will be gone
- Lack of accessibility – refusing to adapt office for clients with physical challenges
- Bigotry or discrimination – refusing to work on a client due to race, religion, size, or sexual orientation
- Inappropriate advertising – using a provocative picture in advertising, presenting misleading qualifications
- Inappropriate dual relationships - dating a client
- Violations of laws – practicing from home when it is not allowed without the proper permits
- Violations of confidentiality – name-dropping clients, telling a spouse details about their partner's session, discussing a massage with a client in a public place such as a grocery store
- Ignoring contraindications – treating a client when the therapist is sick or infectious, ignoring signs or conditions that preclude physical contact
- Informed consent violations - working on a minor without parental knowledge, treating an injury without permission

---

A therapist needs parental permission or permission from a legal guardian before working on a minor.

D. The Therapeutic Relationship

What is **in** the Professional Therapeutic Relationship:
- Confidentiality
- Scope of practice
- Client-centered actions and words
- Consistency
- Informed consent & right of refusal
- Contract
- Rights as professionals

What is **out** of the Professional Therapeutic Relationship:
- Medical advice
- Social needs
- Personal needs
- Spiritual advice
- Psychological counseling
- Other business deals

Informed consent - an agreement to participate in an activity after the purpose has been explained, a protection process for the consumer

Client's right of refusal - a client can stop treatment at any time, a client can refuse any part of treatment even if permission had been given previously

---

Therapist's right of refusal - a therapist can refuse to work on a client in certain situations that make the therapist uncomfortable such as a client with an infectious disease such as hepatitis

Rights as professionals – professionals being clear about what is expected from clients

Power differential - the relationship when an experienced therapist with a PhD performs a massage on a new therapist, or when a recently licensed therapist works under the supervision of a more experienced professional

While on the massage table, a client may be reluctant to make special requests from the therapist due to the power differential.

A power differential may make a therapist reluctant to communicate effectively with a client if the therapist feels the client is more powerful.

If a client reenacts abuse while on the massage table by crying and shaking, the therapist should be calm and accepting.

Gender issues are most likely involved when a client makes a decision based on whether the therapist is male or female.
Gender issues - a male client requesting a female bodyworker

The influence of age on touch is most likely to be a consideration regarding geriatric massage.

Cultural influences are a consideration regarding touch when giving chair massages at an international airport for foreign tourists.

E. Dual Relationships

Dual relationships:
- Assuming two roles with the same person
- When personal and professional roles overlap
- Having a client who is a friend, family member, associate, employee, or supervisor
- Another example of a dual role is when a therapist sells products to a client

Conditions that prompt dual relationships:
- Socializing
- Group affiliation
- Friendship
- Dating
- Sexual activity
- Family
- Bartering
- Client/practitioner reversal
- Employment
- Interactions between students and school personnel

Examples of dual relationship issues:
- A health care professional loses a client after referring them to a massage therapist friend
- A therapist hires a client to do renovations then is disappointed in the work
- A client offers to walk a therapist's dog in exchange for massages, but while the dog is with the client, the dog is injured
- A therapist agrees to exchange massages for artwork to be completed in the future
- A therapist treats a friend and the friend is disappointed with the results
- A teacher and a massage school student start dating and it leads to gossip and tension
- A teacher hires a massage school student as a babysitter and end up getting upset with each other

F. Sexual Misconduct

Sexual misconduct – any action of verbalization of an inappropriate
sexual nature towards a client

Inappropriate behavior from clients:
- Sexual innuendos
- Provocative jokes
- Aggression

Unethical behavior from therapists in a professional relationship:
- Sexual talk
- Sexual relations
- Sexual acts and activities
- Sexual pleasures
- Sexual intercourse
- Being involved in a sexual manner

Sexual misconduct boundary violations:
- Seductive or sexually demeaning gestures, comments, or
  expressions
- Failure to ensure a client's privacy
  - Improper draping
  - Not providing a gown
  - Watching a client undress
- Sexual comments about the client's body
- Sexual jokes
- Strong interest in or disapproval of client's sexual orientation
- Comments about sexual performance
- Conversations about sexual preferences or fantasies

Misconduct involving sexual contact:
- Encouraging the client to masturbate
- Masturbation by the practitioner
- Intercourse
- Inappropriate work
  - Touching breasts for non-therapeutic reasons
  - Inappropriate intra-anal adjustments
- Rape

Sexual harassment:
- A demand for sexual favors in exchange for job benefits
- Hostile work environment including unwelcome acts or visual
  displays

Possibility of inadvertent sexual response during massage:
- Stimulation of nerves in lumbar and sacral plexuses can stimulate nerves in genitals
- Parasympathetic nervous system (rest and digest) provides link between touch and sexual response
- Touch influences the limbic system, which controls emotional and sexual experiences

If sexual arousal occurs during a massage, the practitioner must establish and maintain appropriate boundaries.

Addressing erections in clients:
- If the client shows no signs of discomfort and the therapist is comfortable, it is not necessary to talk about it
- If the client shows signs of discomfort, the therapist should consider talking to the client
- If the client displays sexual intent, the therapist is obligated to talk to the client and intervene

Providing a safe experience for clients:
- Clarify intentions toward clients
- Maintain professional appearance and demeanor
- Establish a professional treatment space
- Provide informed consent
- Choose appropriate music
- Allow privacy for client while changing
- Use appropriate language
- Use appropriate draping
- Be mindful of body contact during session
- Diffuse any hints or signs of sexual arousal
- Keep accurate records of questionable events
- Inform clients of their rights
- Treat all clients equally
- Continuing education in ethics

Professional classifications of touch:
- Appropriate or inappropriate touch
- Therapeutic touch is appropriate touch
- Sexual touch is inappropriate touch

Hostile touch - sexual touch from a professional bodyworker to a client

If a caller asks if the massage includes sex or a client asks to be touched in a sexual manner or for a happy ending, remain professional and explain the services.

If a new client has been asked to get under the covers and the therapist enters the room to find the client naked and on top of the covers, the therapist should leave the room and ask the client to get under the covers.

If a new client mentions that a prior therapist made sexual advances, the therapist should contact the prior therapist to discuss the matter if the therapist knows the prior therapist.

G. Massage / Bodywork-Related Laws and Regulations

State and local governments:
- State and local licensing requirements can be found from state and local government web sites such as the department of licensing
- Licensing is typically done at the state government level
- Laws may restrict the titles that can be used and the scope of practice
- Local governments may have restrictions on what type of business can be conducted from a home and may require a permit
- Local governments control zoning

Licensing and credentialing:
- Licensing is not the same as credentialing
- Licensing means that a government has determined that an individual has met the requirements for a license
- Unlicensed people who practice break the law
- Registration is a means for a government agency to keep track of practitioners
- Credentialing means that an association has determined that an individual meets the requirements for the credentials

If a therapist is aware of someone practicing massage therapy without a license, the therapist should send a complaint to the state's massage board.

H. Scope of Practice

Scope of practice:
- Service limits and boundaries as determined by legal, educational, competency, and accountability factors
- Knowledge base and practice parameters of a profession

Assessment:
- Gathering information to make informed decisions about treatment
- Assessments are within the scope of practice of a massage therapist
- Example - observing where muscles are tight

Diagnosis:
- Assigning a name or label to a group of signs or symptoms
- A diagnosis is outside the scope of practice of a massage therapist
- A diagnosis is usually made by the primary care provider

If a therapist cannot assess a condition, the client should be told to consult their primary care provider about the condition.

Prescribing treatment is outside the scope of practice of a massage therapist.
Soft tissue manipulation is within the scope of practice of a massage therapist.
Giving psychological advice on how to solve personal problems is outside the scope of practice.

If a client asks for advice on what herbs to take to replace prescription medication, the therapist should advise the client to consult with their primary care provider before stopping to take any prescription medication.

If a client tells the therapist that the client is going to stop taking medication or stop medical treatment, the therapist should tell the client to consult their primary care provider.

Refer the client to another professional if the client needs a treatment outside the scope of practice.

I. Professional Communication

Verbal and Nonverbal Communication Skills

Rapport - the development of relationship based on mutual trust and harmony

Communication skill – ability to communicate effectively, therapist's ability to communicate with clients regarding goals, treatments, and outcomes

The most important quality for therapeutic massage and bodywork professionals is caring.

It would be appropriate for the therapist to tell the client that the therapist has a cold, but not appropriate to discuss financial issues, gossip, or personal issues.

When a client discusses personal matters with the therapist, the therapist should just listen and be compassionate.

Communication with the client is the best way to gauge if pressure is appropriate.

Effective communication leads to better quality work, client retention, and referrals.

When a therapist communicates by making a comment about a client's tense muscles, the therapist needs to make sure the comment does not make the client feel put down and humiliated.

If a therapist makes a mistake, it is important to treat the client with respect and admit the mistake.

If a therapist notices a client grimacing in pain while saying that the pressure is fine, the therapist should recognize the nonverbal communication and reduce the pressure.

An example of the need for proactive communication is that a therapist should communicate a policy of charging for missed appointments before actually billing a client for one.

A therapist needs to use a direct communication approach if a client is asking for personal information that the therapist does not want to share, such as a home phone number.

Client Interviewing Techniques

Listening is an important interviewing technique.

If a new client asks the therapist if the therapist is married, the therapist should not share personal information.

If a client feels treated as an object than a person while waiting and filling out forms, it is more important for the therapist to demonstrate sincere and clear communication during the interview.

If a therapist asks about the client's sex life during the interview, the therapist has crossed a boundary.

Communicating with Other Health Professionals

Networking - mutually beneficial business relationships, developing personal and professional contacts for sharing information

When to Refer Clients to Other Health Professionals

Referral - recommendation to see a specific professional
The most appropriate method for giving a referral is to provide a list of practitioners.

Refer the client to a primary care provider immediately if a client comes in with enlarged lymph nodes.

Refer the client to a primary care provider if a client's pulse is strong on one side of the body and weak on the other.

If a client constantly complains about stress and other people's problems, suggest the client seek counseling for the stress.

J. Confidentiality

Confidentiality - keeping information private, respect for client's right to privacy

Therapists should not discuss massage therapy sessions with clients in public.

Therapists should not initiate discussions about massage with clients in public places such as the grocery store or restaurants.

Confidentiality is at the core of professional relationships.

Confidentiality begins with the first phone call and continues for the entirety of the relationship.

Nothing a clients says or does, and no information about a client should be revealed to others without the client's consent, unless disclosure is required by law or a court order, or is necessary for the protection of the public

If a therapist tells everyone the name of a famous person who is a client without the client's permission, the therapist has violated the client's confidentiality.

It would be not be appropriate for the therapist to talk to the client about other clients, for example, the therapist should not provide requested information about a client's former partner or about another client that was seen in the office.

HIPPA – Health Insurance Portability and Accountability Act, enacted in 1996, involves security and privacy of health care issues, specific guidelines that relate to privacy

Disclosure – the sharing of personal information with permission

K. Principles

Standards of practice - rules and procedures for professional conduct and quality of care to be followed by members of a profession, guiding principles by which professionals should conduct themselves and their day-to-day business

Accountability - the quality of accepting the consequences of one's actions

Professionalism - the standard of conduct, goals, and qualities of workers in the same field

Continuing education – supports professional ethics by promoting a higher standard in the profession

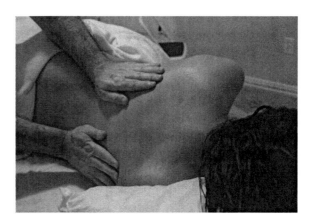

VIII. Guidelines for Professional Practice

A. Proper and Safe Use of Equipment and Supplies

Massage tables:
- Loading capacity - 300 to 450 pounds or more
- Width - 27 to 30 inches
- Length - about 72 inches (6 feet) to 76 inches
- Padding – about 1 to 2 inches of high density foam

Massage table height:
- Determined by therapist's height
- Middle of therapist's thighs
- Hands flat on table while standing straight
- Discomfort in low back – table probably too low
- Discomfort in upper back, shoulders, or arms – table probably too high

Massage environment:
- Massage room minimum 10 feet by 12 feet
- Indirect or natural light
- Soothing music
- 72 to 74 degrees
- Proper ventilation

Lubricants (oils, creams, and lotions):
- Reduce friction and increase comfort
- Oils degrade with heat
- Store in closed contamination-proof dispensers and container
- Never remove lubricants from jar-type containers directly with the fingers

A massage mat is the safest equipment for massaging a 6-month old baby.

The maximum number of beats per minute for music to activate a soothing, relaxing response is 60 beats per minute.

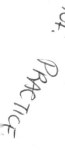

Disinfectants:
- Bleach
  - Sodium hypochlorite
  - 10% solution for disinfecting surfaces and implements
  - Used in laundry for linens and towels
- Ethyl alcohol
  - 70% solution for sanitizing electrodes and implements
  - Mild alcohol solution can be used as rinse to sanitize hands
- Cresol (Lysol®)
  - 1% to 5% solution
  - Used to disinfect floors, sinks and restrooms

B. Therapist Hygiene

CDC Handwashing Recommendations:
- Wash hands after gloves are removed
- Wet hands and apply liquid soap or clean bar soap
- Use plain non-antimicrobial soap
- Rub hands vigorously for at least one minute
- Rinse well and dry hands with disposable towel

> Wash and sanitize hands with soap and warm water between client contacts.

If there is cause for suspicion of bacterial contamination, a mild alcohol solution can be used to rinse the hands.

C. Sanitation and Cleanliness

Levels of Decontamination for Removing Pathogens:
1. Sterilization – most complete process that destroys all living organisms including bacterial spores
   a. Used for surgical instruments in hospitals
2. Disinfection – second level of decontamination, nearly as effective as sterilization but does not destroy bacterial spores
   a. Examples of disinfectants include phenols (Lysol®), chlorine bleach, and ethyl alcohol
3. Sanitation – third level of decontamination generally done with soap and water
   a. Hand washing is an example of sanitation

Universal Precautions for Infection Control:
- Handwashing with soap and water is mandatory before and after contact with every client
- Gloves must be worn if the therapist's skin is not intact
- Gloves should be worn if there is potential for contact with blood or bodily fluids
- Hands must be washed after removing gloves
- Linens soiled with blood or bodily fluids must be gathered and placed in a leakproof bag for transportation to the laundry
- Bleach should be added to the wash for contaminated linens
- Cleaning of walls, floor, and surfaces should be done using products that are effective for sanitation

Standard precautions for preventing transmission of pathogens:
- Proper hand hygiene
- Proper sanitation procedures
- Proper disposal techniques

Sheets:
- Soiled sheets in a hamper, clean sheets off the floor in a closed cabinet
- Linens and towels laundered in hot water with bleach and dried in a hot dryer
- If a therapist drops a sheet on the floor during a massage, the therapist should put the sheet in a hamper and wash the hands
- The CDC states that linens are to be handled in a manner that prevents skin and mucous exposure
- For contaminated sheets sent to a facility that does not use universal precautions, use a biohazard label or red container
- For sheets with blood stains, no label needed if universal precautions are used
- Rancid sheets should be discarded

Infection Precautions:
- Precautions are designed to prevent blood and other secretions from entering practitioner's body
- Hand washing with soap is the primary infection precaution
- The use of gloves is a secondary infection precaution
- Tables and other surfaces contaminated with blood can be sanitized with a 10% bleach solution
- Linens can be disinfected by washing in hot water with detergent and bleach and drying in a hot dryer

Organisms that can cause disease in other organisms:
- Pathogen
- Pathogenic microorganism
- Germs

Examples of infectious diseases:
- Athlete's foot
- HIV
- Hepatitis B

A Hepatitis B vaccination must be made available within 10 days for employees with occupational exposure.

D. Safety Practices

Facilities

Housekeeping/Sanitation:
- Keep all halls and walkways clear
- Keep all carpets vacuumed and sanitized
- Keep all solid floors cleaned and sanitized
- Sanitize all restrooms and bathing facilities
- Make sure all floors in wet areas are slip proof
- Sanitize all equipment surfaces that come in contact with clients including table surfaces, linens, applicators, and vibrators
- Disinfect hydrotherapy tubs, steam cabinets, shower stalls, and wet tables between each use
- Maintain handwashing facilities including germicidal soap, sanitary or paper towels, and a clean and sanitary area
- Commercially launder linens or wash in hot water with bleach and dry in a hot dryer
- Store clean linens in a closed cabinet and soiled linens in a closed container or stored outside the massage room

Equipment:
- Check all equipment for safety and stability including tables, stools, and chairs
- Check all table locks and hinges for stability
- Maintain all equipment including electrical cords and lubrication
- Store equipment and linens properly

Fire safety:
- Maintain functioning smoke and carbon dioxide detectors
- Be familiar with location of fire extinguishers
- Clearly indicate fire exits
- Be aware of evacuation procedures
- Establish a policy regarding the use of open flames, candles and incense
- Contact local fire department for fire safety inspection

First Aid:
- Keep maintained first aid kit on premises
- Make sure all personnel know location of first aid kit
- Staff should learn first aid and CPR
- Emergency information should be in plain view

Heat and ventilation:
- Maintain heat and ventilation systems regularly
- Auxiliary heating devices
  - Use only UL-approved
  - Regularly inspect
  - Turn off when not in use

Client safety:
- Understand paths of infection and use sanitary practices
  - Use clean linens with each client
  - Wash hands before and after each client
  - Provide sanitary bathing facilities and restrooms
  - Avoid open wounds and sores
  - Do not practice massage when sick or contagious
- Provide safe and clear entryways and passages
  - Keep walkways clear and well lighted
  - Provide nonskid walkways and floors
- Assist clients on and off the massage table
- Check to make sure clients are not allergic to products used
- Use proper procedures when dealing with illness and injury, and refer to proper medical authorities when conditions indicate
- Do no harm

Therapist personal safety:
- Use proper body mechanics when lifting and practicing massage to prevent muscle strain and overuse injuries
- Use equipment and modalities properly
- Maintain current first aid and CPR certification
- Know the location of the first aid kit
- Wash hands before and after every treatment
- Know contraindications and only perform therapy within scope of practice
- Give contact information to an associate when performing in-house massage

First Aid

Order of the first aid emergency action steps:
1. Check
2. Call
3. Care

First step when responding to a first aid emergency:
Check the scene and the victim

First aid care when a person is not breathing or unconscious:
Tilt the head back and lift the chin

First step when administering first aid after a person has had a heart attack: Have the person stop activity and rest

First Aid Kit Items:
- Hydrocortisone -treat an external rash
- Antiseptic - clean a wound
- Antibiotic - used against infection
- Aspirin - used for symptoms of a heart attack

E. Therapist Care

Protecting the hands:
- Avoid excessive wrist angles by staying behind massage movements rather than in front of them
- Avoid hyperextending the wrist and using the heel of the hand when applying compression
- Use the forearm and elbows to apply deep pressure
- Use the palmar side of the thumb and fingers rather than the fingertips when applying pressure

---

Practitioner Body Mechanics

- Uses leverage and structural alignment to prevent fatigue
- Observation of body postures in relation to safe and efficient movement
- Increase strength and power available in a movement
- Reduce risk of potential injury to practitioner

Repetitive stress injury - the result of movement by a therapist to the point of damage

---

Reducing the strain on the neck – keep the head up and the shoulders down and relaxed

Symmetric stance (horse stance):
- Therapist facing the massage table with the toes in a line, pointed forward
- Best stance for petrissage

Asymmetric stance (archer stance):
- Therapist has one foot in front of the other with the back foot laterally rotated
- Best stance for deep effleurage
- The angle between the humerus and the side of the body should not exceed how many 90 degrees

Component of wellness:
- Sleep
- Nutrition
- Breathing
- Relaxation
- Exercise
- Stretching

Basic Nutrition Principles

Proteins - classes of complex nitrogen compounds that yield amino acids when hydrolyzed
Carbohydrates - chemical substances includes sugars and starches that only contain carbon, hydrogen, and oxygen
Vitamins and minerals - essential nutrients that can serve as coenzymes or cofactors in an essential metabolic process
Amino Acids - building blocks of protein
Enzymes - organic catalysts that change the rate of a chemical reaction
Glucose - a simple sugar that is the end-product of carbohydrate digestion

Vitamins:
- Vitamin A:
  - Found in butter, egg yolks and yellow vegetables, fat-soluble, formed within the body from alpha, beta, and gamma carotene
  - Deficiency would interfere with growth and reduce immunity
- Vitamin B complex:
  - Found in brewer's yeast, water-soluble
  - Thiamine, Niacin and Riboflavin
  - Necessary for the formation of red blood cells
  - Deficiency would result in digestive disturbances, enlargement of the liver, and disturbance of the thyroid
  - Deficiency of Thiamine would cause beriberi
- Vitamin C -
  - Found in citrus fruits, water-soluble
- Vitamin D:
  - Found in milk, fat-soluble
  - Necessary for the absorption of calcium and phosphorus
  - Synthesized within the body by ultraviolet radiation
- Vitamin E:
  - Strong anti-oxidant and immune supporter, fat-soluble
  - The general population has no deficiency
- Vitamin K:
  - Found in fats, grains, and fishmeal, regulates blood coagulation, made within the body, fat-soluble
  - Deficiency prolongs blood-clotting time and causes bleeding

For growing children and pregnant women, it is recommended to include more minerals in the diet.

Minerals:
- Sodium and potassium - required by nerve cells and muscle cells to conduct electricity
- Magnesium and zinc - nutrients that the body requires an extremely small amount to function normally
- Calcium and magnesium - critical for proper muscle contraction
- Zinc - an essential nutrient involved in most metabolic pathways
- Magnesium - component of enzymes required for synthesis of ATP
- Iron - necessary for hemoglobin
- Calcium - helps in the formation of teeth and bones

Insoluble carbohydrates add bulk to food and help with bowel movements.

Animal proteins have a great variety of amino acids.

Recommended calorie distribution for healthy eating:
Less than 30% of calories from fats, 50%-60% carbohydrates, 12%-15% proteins

Recommended number of servings per day:
- Bread, cereal, rice, and pasta group - 6 to 11 servings
- Vegetable group - 3 to 5 servings
- Fruit group - 3 to 5 servings
- Milk, yogurt and cheese group - 2 to 3 servings
- Meat, poultry, fish, dried beans, and nuts group - 2 to 3 servings
- Fats, oils, and sweets group - use sparingly

Daily Needs:
- 2 to 3 liters of water
- 1,600 to 2,800 calories
- 45 to 63 grams of protein

F. Draping

Draping - keeping a client covered during the massage
Warmth, modesty, client's comfort, establish trust, client feels safe

Avoid light, see-through colors when draping.

Top cover method:
- A table covering along with a top covering
- Large enough to cover the entire body
- Large bath sheet towel or half of a full or double sheet
- Minimum size for top cover 72 inches long and 36 inches wide

Full sheet draping:
- Uses a full size double flat sheet to cover the table and the client
- Minimum width 80 inches

Any materials coming in contact with the client's skin must be freshly laundered and sanitary.

Clean linens must be used for each client.

A common method for draping:
1. The therapist instructs the client to remove clothing and lay on the table covered with the drape
2. The therapist leaves the room
3. The client disrobes, gets on the table, and covers themselves with the drape

G. Business Practices

Basic Business and Accounting Practices

Business plan - a road map to achieve goals
Financial records - include numbers such as income and expenses
Balance sheet - shows assets and liabilities
Resume - a one-page document that includes the career objective
Word of mouth - best advertising for a massage therapist
Marketing - promoting the business by methods such as brochures, business cards, or donated services
Management – running a business including maintaining the office, keeping a budget, monitoring income and expenses, and verifying credentials
Overhead – fixed expenses such as monthly rent
Net income – profit, based on gross income minus expenses
Start-up costs - the initial costs of beginning a business such as the cost of obtaining credentials and a business license
Barter income – revenue from trade of which 100% must be 100% must be reported to the IRS
Gross income - the sum of fees collected
Mission statement - a statement of goals and purpose of a business
Media - systems of mass communication
Business cards - a simple way to provide contact information
Brochures - a way to explain services in detail to prospective clients including information on types of massage, qualifications, and fees
Insurance billing - the 97000 series is the code for massage therapy

Regulations Pertaining to Income Reporting

Income that must be reported to the IRS:
• Wages
• Barter income (100%)
• Tips

Revenue from a gift certificate is reportable as income when it is purchased.

Business expenses such as the cost of equipment, linens, business clothes, business cards, advertising, licensing, insurance, memberships, and continuing education are tax deductible.

IRS Forms:
- Form 1099-B - barter exchange transactions
- Form 1099-MISC - fees for subcontractors recorded
- Form 4562 - depreciation
- Form 2106 - employee business expenses
- Schedule K-1 of Form 1065-B - partner's share of income or loss
- Schedule C of Form 1040 - the net profit from a business
- Form W-2 – wages reported on from prepared by employer and provided to employees

Barter exchange - an organization with members who trade services

Need for Liability Insurance

Liability insurance:
- Protects against lawsuits
- General premise liability insurance - protects against slips and falls
- Professional liability insurance -protects against malpractice and claims of professional misconduct
- Product liability insurance - protects against an adverse reaction to a lotion
- Liability can be limited by keeping accurate records

Property Insurance:
- Protects against monetary loss for damage to a building or equipment
- Includes premises fire damage insurance or renters insurance

Additional insured endorsement - typically requested by an employer or landlord

Legal defense coverage - pays attorney's fees

Legal Entities (e.g., Independent Contractor, Employee)

Sole proprietorship - a business with one owner who is the only employee
Partnership - a company with two or more persons with ownership and personal liability, a relationship between two or more persons to carry on a trade or business

Limited Liability Corporation (LLC) - similar to a corporation but with the partners having limited personal liability

Corporation - a business arrangement with one or more owners and limited liability

DBA - the doing business as name

S-Corporation - avoids double taxation

Taxes an S corporation is liable for:
- Income tax
- Estimated tax
- Employment tax

Advantages of being self-employed:
- Work on own schedule, more flexible hours
- Keep greater portion of fees collected

Disadvantages of being self-employed:
- Less steady income than being an employee
- Responsible for own taxes
- Must pay for own facilities and supplies

Employee - working in an established place of business with the hours set by the employer, paid by the hour or on commission, receive W2 forms from employer

Advantages of being an employee:
- The employer provides the facilities and supplies
- Steady paycheck
- Can focus more on massage

Disadvantages of being an employee:
- Keep less of fees collected
- Less flexible hours

Independent contractor – working like an employee while being self-employed, setting own hours, paid by the hour or on commission, files own taxes

About the Author

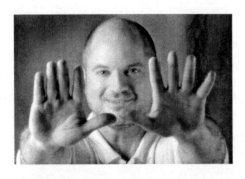

Philip Martin McCaulay is the President of Medical Massage Care Authority LLC and a graduate of Bodymechanics School of Myotherapy and Massage in Olympia, Washington. His other massage publications include <u>Medical Massage Care's Therapeutic Massage National FSMTB Massage & Bodywork Licensing Examination MBLEx Practice Exams 2010 Edition</u>, <u>Medical Massage Care's Therapeutic Massage National Certification Practice Exams 2008 Edition</u> and <u>Medical Massage Care's Therapeutic Massage National Certification Exam Study Guide</u>.

Martin has also written and published practice exam books and study guides for licensing and certification exams in the pension, investment, finance, and real estate fields. With a B.A. in Mathematics from Indiana University, Martin is a Fellow of the Society of Actuaries (FSA), a Fellow of the Conference of Consulting Actuaries (FCA), a Member of the American Academy of Actuaries (MAAA), and an Enrolled Actuary (EA). Martin serves on the Education and Examination Committee of the Society of Actuaries.

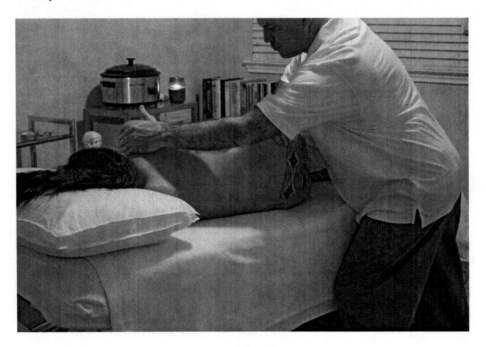

Reference List

Ashley, Martin. *Massage: A Career at Your Fingertips*. 3rd Edition. Barrytown, New York: Station Hill Press, 1998

Benjamin, Ben and Cherie Sohnen-Moe. *The Ethics of Touch*. Tucson: Sohnen-Moe Associates, Inc., 2004.

Beck, Mary F. *Theory and Practice of Therapeutic Massage*. 4th Edition. Clifton Park, New York: Thompson Delmar Learning, 2006.

Biel, Andrew. *Trail Guide to the Body*. 3rd Edition. Boulder, Colorado: Books of Discovery, 2005.

Braun, Mary Beth and Stephanie Simonson. *Introduction to Massage Therapy*. Baltimore: Lippincott Williams and Wilkins, 2005.

Clemente, Carmine. *Anatomy: A Regional Atlas of the Human Body*. 4th Edition. Baltimore: Lippincott Williams and Wilkins, 1997.

Fritz, Sandy. *Fundamentals of Therapeutic Massage*. 3rd Edition. St. Louis: Mosby, 2004.

Fritz, Sandy and M. James Grosenbach. *Essential Sciences for Therapeutic Massage: Anatomy, Physiology, Biomechanics and Pathology*. 2nd Edition. St. Louis: Mosby, 2004.

Kendall, Florence Peterson, Elizabeth Kendall McCreary, Patricia Geise Provance, Mary McIntyre Rodgers, and William Anthony Romani. *Muscles: Testing and Function with Posture and Pain*. 5th Edition. Baltimore: Lippincott Williams and Wilkins, 2005.

McIntosh, Nina. *The Educated Heart: Professional Boundaries for Massage Therapists, Bodyworkers, and Movement Teachers.* 2nd Edition. Baltimore: Lippincott Williams and Wilkins, 2005.

Premkumar, Kalyani. *The Massage Connection: Anatomy and Physiology*. 2nd Edition. Baltimore: Lippincott Williams and Wilkins, 2004.

Rattay, Fiona and Linda Ludwig. *Clinical Massage Therapy: Understanding, Assessing and Treating Over 70 Conditions*. Ontario: Talus, Inc., 2000.

Salvo, Susan. *Massage Therapy: Principles and Practices*. Philadelphia: W.B. Saunders Company, 1999.

Sohnen-Moe, Cherie. *Business Mastery*. 3rd Edition. Tucson: Sohnen-Moe Associates, Inc., 2005.

Tappan, Frances M. and Patricia J. Benjamin. *Handbook of Healing Massage Techniques*. 4th Edition. Connecticut: Appleton and Lange, 2005.

Thomas, C.L., ed. *Taber's Cyclopedic Medical Dictionary*. 19th Edition. Philadelphia: Davis Co., 2001.

Thompson, Diana L. *Hands Heal, Communication, Documentation, and Insurance Billing for Manual Therapists*. 3rd Edition. Baltimore: Lippincott Williams and Wilkins, 2006.

Tortora, Gerald, and Sandra Reynolds Grabowski. *Principles of Anatomy and Physiology*. 10th Edition. New York: Harper and Collins Publishers, Inc., 2004.

Werner, Ruth. *A Massage Therapist's Guide to Pathology*. 2nd Edition. Baltimore: Lippincott Williams and Wilkins, 2002.

Wible, Jean. *Pharmacology for Massage Therapy*. Baltimore: Lippincott Williams and Wilkins, 2005.

LaVergne, TN USA
13 June 2010
185978LV00003B/18/P

9 781449 505998